THIN & BLESSED

THE ANSWER TO WEIGHT LOSS
IS ALREADY INSIDE YOU

THIN &
BLESSED

*10 Wise Decisions for
Love, Power, & Joy*

ELIZABETH
BRICKMAN

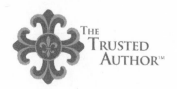

THE
TRUSTED
AUTHOR™

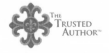

THE 10 WISE DECISIONS OF THIN & BLESSED

1st Decision: I WILL FINISH

2nd Decision: I WILL LIVE LIFE LOVED

3rd Decision: I WILL HAVE A THIN IDENTITY

4th Decision: I WILL FORGET

5th Decision: I WILL FLEX

6th Decision: I WILL FORSAKE

7th Decision: I WILL MAKE IT FUN

8th Decision: I WILL FAST

9th Decision: I WILL FINESSE

10th Decision: I WILL FORGE

CONTENTS

"Do not go where the path may lead,
go instead where there is no path and leave a trail."
—Ralph Waldo Emerson

DEDICATION

I dedicate THIN & BLESSED *to every overweight person
who yearns to be thin.*

You have my respect and my love.

*This is the book I myself needed to read.
I have written it for you.*

*"God has given each of you some special abilities;
be sure to use them to help each other,
passing on to others God's many kinds of blessings."*
(1 Peter 4:10)

THANKS AND ACKNOWLEDGMENTS

O h, the power of words! Johanna Fox Turner, you spoke one unforgettable sentence that set my author-resolve into steel. Bobbie Wolgemuth, your loving personal advice, "Write to *one* woman," is on *every* page. I'll thank you in heaven one day. Diane Hampton, I've never met you but I want to hug you. Andrea Barberis, your words changed the course of my weight, my health, and my life. Debra Austin, your creative excellence has made exercise a joy! *"Little Vanessa"* Delgado, my smart, talented assistant, thanks for your *big* talent, loving values and enduring commitment. Jeannie Evans, Roz Belliveau, thank you for urging me to pursue thin, as impossible as it then seemed. Eva Marie Everson, thank you for extraordinary leadership and for writing fictional characters I love like friends. Robin Joss, thanks for being my accountability partner. Glenda Shambo, Joan Cox, Miriam Duame, Lossi Lacoste, and Lupe Padilla, thank you for *modeling thin.* Jean Siegal, Trina Romeo, thanks for reading my entire, unedited manuscript. *Your feedback thrilled me.* Esther Braglia, my 87-year-old mother, you are an excellent proof-reader. Andrew Mackay, VP Publishing Services, BelieversPress, you gave more of yourself than any author could ask. Your dedication is inspiring; your counsel smart, wise, skilled, and relevant. Thank you for being there for me.

And thank you, Guy, for your steadfast love. You are *more*

than my husband. You are my friend, my lover, *my life*. First, last, and always, it is you, my beloved.

Thanks to all my family, on earth *and in heaven*. I love you.

☙

I thank God for his decision to send Jesus Christ to save the world. Thank you, Lord!

THE JOYFUL BEGINNING

After I made the decision to become *thin*, I braced myself, knowing from experience what to expect: the chronic irritation of hunger, the angst of the scale not budging, the overwhelming desire for forbidden food, the raging, internal fight between the good me and the bad me, the dread of exercise, and the frustrating over-focus on food.

Thankfully, I did not get what I expected.

I did not expect *joy*. Not on a weight-loss endeavor. So I dismissed it. But *joy* kept showing up, again and again—a different kind of joy originating from a different place inside me.

How could this be? My life, like yours, is full of its share of stresses and overloads. My workday is pocked by minor, but infuriating, irritants. Tension is not a stranger, nor is sleeplessness.

But there it was: *joy*—palpable, endorphin-like joy. It was an undercurrent that presented itself to my senses daily, oddly interrupting my responsibly distracted inner life.

The 10 Wise Decisions, I began to realize, had put me on a kind of joyride—a joyride to *thin*.

A joyride to thin? Is that anything like a joyride to a root canal?

I was soon to discover that joy is more than a byproduct of the 10 Wise Decisions.

Joy is its compass.

My present weight is lower than my fantasy goal—something I never dreamed possible. The 10 Wise Decisions lovingly surrounded me and *they escorted me to thin.*

> *Joy is more than a byproduct of the 10 decisions. Joy is its compass.*

I am now riding through life in the *thin* lane. Just as a lane on a highway, it's a narrow lane, a safe lane, well defined with white stripes on either side to help remind me where I want to be. Written on those reassuring stripes are my 10 Wise Decisions, which gently affirm my destination. I eagerly stay within them. Free to change lanes to meet today's weakness or emphasis, my daily accountability sounds a warning if I accidentally veer outside the lane *of my choosing.* Eating well has become a joyous freedom, not a constriction, and I cling to that freedom tightly.

The 10 Wise Decisions have empowered me to be the strong and loving Defender; the Protector of what I permit to go into my body. It makes food beg for entrance into the *loved and sacred* place that belongs to me.

Meals are delightful now, *free of conflict and angst,* chosen each day out of a strong, *God-fident* identity. I say *yes* to any food that makes me feel powerful, confident, and holy. When I say *no,* I feel triumphant, not terrible; delighted, not deprived.

Thin has been an easy and natural consequence of my 10 Wise Decisions; something I don't have to worry about or even talk about. I feel like I've gotten my life back—*my real life*.

No longer conflicted about the application of my faith to the stewardship of my body, I have peace. Peace in my closet, peace with photos and mirrors, peace meeting new friends, peace reconnecting with old ones. I am surely THIN & BLESSED.

And so I present to you *a different kind of plan* that leads to *a different kind of thin*—a thin that is *identity-based* and *empowerment-driven*. The 10 Wise Decisions deliver you to a *secure and relaxed* kind of thin, achievable with a remarkable absence of pain. Here you'll find no sorrow.

Decision 1 will surge your unstoppable purpose.
Decision 2 will fill your empty heart with love.
Decision 3 will establish your truest identity.
Decision 4 will cancel your un-thin past.
Decision 5 will build new power and amazing confidence.
Decision 6 will lead you to diet mercies.
Decision 7 will celebrate and inspire fun.
Decision 8 will break your bondage to food.
Decision 9 will creatively outsmart interference.
Decision 10 will design a personal plan to get and *stay* thin!

I know that weight-loss plans generally ask you to adhere to a prescribed plan. But I'll show you how to *make it up yourself*. At the end of each chapter, I'll invite you to sign and date your decision, to *affirm it is now your own*.

⚜

Thin is personal. Together with your doctor, you will *redefine* it according to criteria unique to you.

I describe myself as thin because, according to my doctor, my exercise physiologist—according to every graph and measurement, my age, frame, height, muscle-mass, BMI, and pant size, I am now classified as thin.

Others of my height and frame are far thinner than I am. I can touch some fat on my hips, and my face is trim, but not gaunt. Your *personal thin* may be size 2. Or you may long for a victory lap at size 12. Thin is an individual assessment. Aside from your physician, it should not be determined for you by others. Your thin belongs to you, not to them.

Ordinary days are no threat to thin. I maintain a low weight and a lean appearance peacefully and without struggle—*without fear or fight.*

In the past, I would lose weight, and *then* try to figure out how to maintain it. I always hoped for the best. But the best is never what I got. Now I live with a sense of completeness, an assurance that I will always be able to maintain my low weight *naturally.* What a gift!

This, dear one, is the book I so needed to read. *And that's why I had to write it for you.*

THE DREAM OF THIN

Y *ou don't have to be thin to be beautiful.* Some of the most gorgeous women I know are *not thin.* You *don't* have to be thin to win the love and favor of God, whose beloved come in all shapes and sizes, including thin and un-thin. Carrying a little extra weight may be fine if your doctor says you're healthy, and if you are happy and comfortable.

Being thin won't make you happy—or so they say. *Well, you could have fooled me!* Oh, becoming thin isn't how you fix a bad marriage or retrain a stubborn child. It isn't how you make your car payment, ease your job worries, or heal from illness or loss.

Then why choose thin? What will it do for you?

Thin will positively and joyfully impact a large number of issues you deal with on a daily basis. I assure you those issues will be happier, sweeter when you are thin. *Thin* casts a wide net over so very many aspects of life. How can you *not* be happier when thin?

Thin isn't the *only* path to increased happiness. But to me, *thin* feels safer. More welcoming. It feels stronger, and not just physically. *Thin* feels more self-contained, *fuller* from the inside-out. Less needy.

Thin isn't everything in life. But I like thin. I like it *way* better than *un-thin*. Thin is a gift for a great life.

Do you have an unstoppable desire to be thin? I know why. And I know how.

I wrestled for a lifetime with frustrating overweight. And then I became THIN & BLESSED by making 10 Wise Decisions about *who I am* and *how I relate to food*. It was *easy, joyful, natural, and fun*. I reached my dream weight. You will, too.

Thin had been my longing, my dream. For me, being *un-thin* was silent torment. My extra girth felt like rocks strung around my neck to form a yoke, keeping me in bondage to an identity I *did not choose* and *did not want*. I grieved, knowing that the un-thin life I was living was a lesser substitute for the thin life I so wanted. Though for years I tried to accept modest overweight as my reasonable standard, I was unable to shake the "*if only*" fantasy of thin, a fantasy that each birthday seemed to pull further away from my reach.

My professional life was filled with earnest achievement; my marriage as tender and loving as any I've seen. In some ways I had the life that others only dream of. But there was a dark shadow cast over my other significant blessings. Overweight had me in its grip, an unrelenting chokehold on my otherwise blessed life. It caused angst and humiliation, shame and remorse.

I looked okay, sort of. Certainly better than I had in earlier years, before some weight had been lost. Like a fluffy hen, I had settled complacently into a lifestyle of only *modest* over-weight. A part of me was actually *proud* that I had managed to come this far. *Proud* that my compulsions were slight com-pared to some others. *Proud* that many un-thin people would beg to have a weight problem as *minor* as mine.

But though fewer than twenty pounds remained in the way of excess, I winced at the very thought of them, because deep down, I knew *exactly why* those defiant pounds were there. Increasingly uncomfortable before God, my weight was a visible contradiction of my sincere beliefs, a maddening dis-traction from all I wanted to do with my life.

Was my dissatisfaction purely about beauty? *No, it was worse.*

What troubled me more was my unwholesome relation-ship with food. I knew there existed a more peaceful way to interact with it; I observed it in my thin friends. They had calmness, an ease in their relationship with food; a rightness, evenness. They had a truer alignment of fork-to-values than was operational in my own life. Were these food-virtues pos-sible for me? Are they possible for you?

I argued. All the time. With myself. *Look how far you've come. You've done so well. At least you've kept most of it off. Your husband is happy. What do you expect, at your age?*

At your age. Oh, that. The inevitability of age.

My ever-rational mind seriously considered surrender-ing to this hopeless struggle. *Why continue wrestling with an impossible dream? Count your other blessings, accept a little overweight and be done with it. The tyranny of food is big-ger than you. How can you ever hope to tackle the impossible dream of thin?*

But some dreams refuse to die. They peek out at unexpected moments.

My emotional heart was divided. It see-sawed between wistfully yearning for thin and scolding itself into a more rational acceptance of what I thought was meant-to-be.

But my spirit knew an unfathomable truth. In that sacred space where words are unformed, I was being gently wooed toward a greater weight victory than I could ever "dare to ask or even dream of" (EPHESIANS 3:20).

The 10 Wise Decisions would soon present themselves to me, decisions that would empower me with riveting emotional newness, spiritual awakening, and the gift of mental strength. These 10 decisions would lead me comfortably, joyfully and naturally to a state I can only describe as THIN & BLESSED.

The 10 wise decisions would empower me with riveting emotional newness, spiritual awakening, and the gift of mental strength.

I had been under an incorrect presumption that the push-pull within me was primarily about *food*. I would soon discover otherwise. My true struggle was about *relationship*—my relationship with myself. And with God. *No wonder that dream had refused to die!*

Have you ever wondered why a person as productive as you, as disciplined as you, as experienced as you, cannot seem to conquer overweight?

Then still trapped, I wondered, too. Overweight had kidnapped my best destiny; I was sure of it. I had lived my life as a hostage of sorts, chained to a food-focused lifestyle I had long ago outgrown. Weight management had been an annoying nag in my life, like a drip you don't even realize is agitating you until somebody finally turns the blasted thing off.

Increasingly restless, I wanted out. I wanted a new life, a new freedom. I wanted to wear new dresses. I wanted to dream new dreams.

Frantically, I reconsidered every diet I'd tried, every weight-loss book I'd read. There just had to be a way to overcome this. Then one day it happened. Though I had no answers yet, I set my will. I found my *no*. I was done.

My deliverance was ushered in through a back door. After a sleepless night, I awoke with a headache, stomachache, and heartache. The gloomy rain outside my kitchen window was no match for the gloom inside me. I opened my prayer journal and wrote this:

Dear Lord,
I don't feel good.
I need to lose weight.
I need to clean out my body of waste and toxins.
I don't know what to do.
I don't know what method to take.
Show me your best and highest route for my life, my
    health, my ministry.
Give me divine and holy protection over the evil one who
    would sabotage me.
Show me the high path and calling. Protect me, heal me.
I want to live healthy, engaged with life.
I want my spirit to prosper.
I need this body. And I'm willing (I think) to get it right
    and to follow direction.
Please, please make clear my best, ordained route to
    body health, healing, and a God-weight.
Please…

Is there a yearning within you today, crying for another chance at thin? Do not fight it, and do not reason against it. Honor it! Honor the cry of your heart, for it may be God calling you to live a more free and victorious lifestyle than you ever dreamed possible.

For what is the real point of thin, anyway? Is it to conform to society's arbitrary standards? *Certainly not.* Or to please a certain audience in your life? *I hope not.* Is it to increase your ego? *I doubt it.*

I have come to believe the dream of *thin* comes from the heart of God, for his purposes. Through its victory, we learn fundamental lessons of personal stewardship. We grow and are strengthened. We increase our sensitivity to sharing his resources for mankind. And maybe best of all, we model our most powerful selves for those we love.

I did not get thin to be beautiful, though I always hoped to be. I got thin because for me, the alternative was too costly, too annoying, and too distracting from my highest destiny. My overweight did not represent my personal best. It did not reflect the excellence I wanted to deliver to the world.

Twelve weeks after I wrote that letter to God came my special day. In the space of a single breath appeared a hazy vision of triumph, of freedom. On that day that I made the first of 10 Wise Decisions … and my whole world changed. That glorious decision formed the first crack in my bondage to food.

Trembling, I sensed that full deliverance was near. Over the next months, I made and completed the 10 Wise Decisions you now hold in your hands. I wrested free of my captor and embarked on a spiritual joyride that delivered me all the way to thin.

I planned my own escape meticulously. *And now I've planned yours.* I don't know why God generously delivered me to thin. But this much I know: he didn't do it *just* for me. With open heart, I trust that as you read these words, your own special day is approaching.

Be alert, dear one. Ready yourself! Grab your pen and highlighter. Reboot your courage. Put on holy armor. Set your will and step up to the plate. The emptier, more sweetly satisfying plate. Your time of transformation is upon you.

Choose this day whom you will serve.

Choose this day *who you will become.*

Are you ready? Let's go...

CAT AND MOUSE
The story of your diets

The playful grey kitten focused intently on her game of catch-the-mouse. Fully engaged, she darted and swiped with passionate paws at the colorful mouse-toy dangling from strings on a wooden stick. Under control by her owner's hand, the toy swayed and bobbed as Kitty excitedly pounced and batted her paws to catch it.

But poor Kitty could not catch her mouse. Enthusiasm ebbed. Frustration built. Fatigue set in; then boredom. Finally, she tired of trying and simply gave up.

Sound familiar? *Isn't it the story of your past diets?* You started a weight loss program. At first, you tried with all your might. You pounced wholeheartedly at the *prize of thin* dangling before you on a string. You pledged your commitment to anyone within earshot. With impressive optimism, you pursued your conquest of the pounds, your lifestyle temporarily shoved aside for the "greater good." You faithfully counted every point, drank every shake, bought every product and did everything asked of you ... and even more.

But the game was unwinnable. Your early passion sank to forced effort, then to stoicism. So much self-denial. So little reward. So much output of your limited energy. Isn't life hard enough? The *dream of thin* had distanced itself ... *again.* It was your unconquerable, life draining nemesis.

But what if we could rewrite your story?

Consider for a moment Kitty. All she really needed to do, *with no additional effort,* was swipe at the *hand controlling the strings.* One good pounce at the right thing—not the mouse, not even the strings, but the hand controlling those strings—would have caused immediate release. Kitty would have joyously won her mouse-reward, and quickly, too, with playful energy intact to savor the spoils of her victory.

We, the *un-thin,* have been swiping for too long at strings being dangled before us: strict diet programs, right foods, wrong foods, right timing, wrong combinations ... just a bunch of strings that string us along. And we never have caught our "mouse." Oh, we've tried. We've given our all. But eventually, we've wearied of these disheartening games. How could we not?

I'm going to take you on a thrilling new joyride to thin.

After a lifetime wrestling with frustrating overweight, I became THIN & BLESSED by simply making 10 Wise Decisions about *who I am* and *how I relate* to food. It was easy, joyful, natural and fun, and my 10 Wise Decisions caused the grip of overweight to release. I reached my dream weight; I caught my mouse. *You will, too.*

You'll eat what *you* want most, from choices based on criteria that *you alone* define and control. *Each wise decision will send shock and awe to every fat cell in your body.* As your weight runs away from you, you'll feel the thrill of an exultant conqueror. Not the misery of a dieter. Shrink with deprivation? Ha! You'll swell with power! The 10 Wise Decisions will cause the grip of overweight to release.

Joy will be your faithful companion. You'll depend on a forgotten friend for big support: *you*. You'll speak powerful, loving truth to yourself, cancel your old, overweight identity, empty yourself of what hasn't worked, and fill yourself with what *does*. You'll forge a tactical new plan, the first one ever that fits perfectly; so pleasing, you'll hope it never ends. You'll fine-tune it to enhance your increasingly blessed and unique life. You'll have fun with playful new games that stimulate your awareness and intention.

I reached my dream weight; I caught my mouse. You will, too.

✧

Will it be different this time? Yes! The path to *thin* is both possible and pleasurable. Even for you. *Especially for you.*

You're going on a joyride, dear one, to a land where small sizes fit perfectly and photos are friendly. Exhilarated, invigorated, you'll reach your destination with energy fully intact to savor your coveted prize. Make no mistake: the prize of *this* game is *thin*.

No matter your past, you can be victorious. The 10 Wise Decisions are far more powerful than that which has controlled your strings. Get ready: the awful grip of overweight is going to surrender and release. *You'll see.*

Your weight struggle is an *old story that needs a new ending*. You deserve to joyously win this time. *And you will!*

Oh yes, dear one. Prepare yourself. You are going to catch your mouse!

A VISION OF THIN

... An exciting look forward

There you are, tagged in a photo a friend posted on Facebook, and oh my, you look really good! Photos no longer have the power to make you wince or ruin your day. Posing is less staged. Everybody assumes you're happier, and you are. The wrestling match between you and your weight has ended, replaced with new happiness and energy. You're having a great time with life!

You've formed a simple, livable framework for a lifestyle of leanness. Designed by you, for you alone, it contains all that you want—and none of what you don't. It royally and deferentially regards your tastes and preferences, your pleasures and radical delights, your schedule, restaurants, beliefs, and even your quirky family.

Your life feels less derailed, more intentional. Not from a new way of *doing*, but from a new way of *thinking—not* diet-based, *not* guilt-based, but *identity-based*. Those who knew you before have a celebratory appreciation of your newfound, thin state of being.

New diet styles and trends are mostly ignored by you, unless of course they happen to meet with your *picky personal approval*. Who's the boss? You are. Not the food. Not your friends. Not any diet. You will never again surrender to anybody else's idea of what is supposed to work for you. All this, plus *thin, too! It's a wow of a change, from the inside out.*

Your appetite has miraculously been tamed, replaced by peace. Food is easy. You modestly intake food—and voraciously intake *life.* You are content, filled with the right stuff. Not overfed with food, but with an abundance of thriving spirit and a brand new sense of self.

You look great, feel strong, and are very much in control of your grown-up choices.

No longer feeling like a helpless child who can't climb over a burdensome wall of weight, you have scaled it nicely, thank you—all the way to the top and gleefully down the other side in a joyride to *thin.* Relaxed and quietly composed, you are finally in charge of *you.* Others have only to look at you to know it. You see it in their faces. Your easy confidence shows them that you know it too.

As a little child you dreamed of the magical grown-up you might one day become. That vision, no longer tarnished by excess weight, has at last been fulfilled. You look great, feel strong, and are very much in control of your grown-up choices. At the same time, you feel blissfully young, with new excitement and a fresh-start attitude about all sorts of things.

The energy around you is now distinctly different. Your presence in the world is neither pretentious nor self-effacing, just quietly assured. Your world is enlarging, with new relationships expanded by your lovely appearance and unhindered by personal compulsion. You walk into a crowded room needing to offer no explanation for your appearance. Confident, you feel you could be introduced to just about anybody, knowing you would not have to overcome their initial assessment based on your size. Your outside finally reflects your inside; it's an authentic outflow of the real you, defining who you really are. So your self-esteem and confidence are less forced, more natural. Social groups no longer disturb you. No one judges *thin*. You feel thankful.

Relationships have been redefined; roles revised. Your personal empowerment stands at an all-time high. You find yourself increasingly respected. The equation is tilting; You feel inexplicably as if you could offer less and yet would receive more from those around you.

But you have no intention to give less. You're ready to give more, far more, out of your new abundance of energy and self-joy. The energy you once needed to hold onto your emotional well-being, is now applied as you deem fit for whatever new opportunity interests you. And a lot of new things interest you. You are one free woman. You are one free man.

At last, you personally experience the headiness and benefits of those who are thin. Pain has been removed from your facial expression, the pain of shame, the pallor of emotional suffering, and the shadow of secrets kept and promises broken. These have been replaced with a new radiance and light from within. Whatever your health status, you feel better, stronger, more vibrant. Smaller, but mightier, that's you.

The world looks prettier, as if you're wearing special glasses that add radiant light. Sometimes it seems like a very good dream. Yet you're quite awake, more than ever before.

And the clothes. *Oh, the clothes!* They glide on and zip up smoothly; a single-digit pants size, a fantasy dress. Fearlessly, you walk into any clothing store, try on what attracts, and it fits. You catch yourself smiling at the fitting room mirror. Unfazed by compliments from the sales clerk, you already know how you look. *And how you look is good.*

Your closet is tidy and orderly, simple and full, efficiently and productively filled with a fabulous wardrobe of items you can actually wear. There is new simplicity in your garment selection and confidence in your appearance. Sure of how you look and who you are, at blessed peace in your small clothing size, you no longer need to spend as much on clothes, and you generously redirect those extra resources outward.

That wedding invitation you receive is no longer tainted by panic or dread. Clothing is a peaceful subject now; the need for it stirs no anxiety. Even if the airline loses your bag, you remain in confident control, knowing you can replace what you need from just about anywhere. Former *"clothing catastrophes"* are reclassified as "minor inconveniences." You are able to shop successfully for small-sized, great-looking, well-fitting garments in any city, in any price range, in any situation you happen to be in.

Your motivation to remain thin arises from a deep sense of *privilege.* You no longer need a strong willpower to remain thin, because you have a strong new identity, one you cherish and protect. Stronger and stronger, each time you say no to that which does not befriend you, you are swept with a new wave of empowerment. Nothing will rob you of your identity again.

With intimacy unobstructed, closeness is increasing between you and the one you love. There is a marked ease of interacting, of moving, even of traveling. And energy? Your well-tuned engine is ready to zoom, zoom, zoom.

Your ministry and service to others are ordered by a right balance of self-care vs. other-centered care. Helping make others strong no longer means weakening you.

I see you at your most beautiful, your most favorite self. And I rejoice with you.

Your joyride to *thin* was gleeful, not torturous. Less about a destination and all about a powerful *new starting place*.

Seeing yourself differently made simple your direction. It was fun and natural. It just felt right. *And maybe for the first time ever, it actually worked.*

> *You no longer need a strong willpower to remain thin.*

For too long, you were like a flowering plant whose identity had been undiscovered, and so was planted out of place. Finally, you have been planted in the right field, where you are blossoming. Sweet is your growth and sweet will it always be.

You didn't do this for anybody else. You did it for you. You had longed for it, imagined it, wished for it, and prayed for it. You wondered if it were possible. Turned out, it was possible. You did it. You finished.

What felt impossible is now laughable. You smile, because now you know the glory of *thin*. You've come home. You have returned to you. From now on, you always will.

You are going to so love being *thin*.

I embrace my Vision of Thin, and to that vision I add the following:

Signature _____ Date _____

Next: Our 1ˢᵗ Wise Decision will send shock and awe to every fat cell in your body!

I WILL FINISH

Once and for all...

One morning I awoke and made the first of 10 Wise Decisions that changed my life. It was a *spectacular* decision that caused the *first crack* in the stronghold of my overweight.

I will finish it. I will get rid of the extra weight, all of it. I am going to enjoy the rest of my life as a thin person.

On that day I was *done with it,* with *all* of it. *Done with dealing with it. Done with feeling the feelings. Done.*

But... *Finish it?* Wasn't that a rather grand pronouncement from one whose weight had plagued her for a lifetime? Wasn't it... a bit *unrealistic?* Finish it. *Sure...* Then what? Climb Mount Everest?

Nonetheless, there was an inexplicable absoluteness in my head. A sense of finality that *defied the logic of the present.* Out of me had arisen a new will, laser-focused on a grand, once-and-for-all finish. My conviction was crystal clear. I would get thin and live like a thin person for the rest of my life. On this, I would be unmovable.

From then on, there would be no wavering, no self-nego-tiating, no wondering. I was *finished* with overweight—*and everything about weight*. And somehow I knew as I trusted the sun to rise, I could trust that I would find a *new* way to solve this very *old* problem.

Did I have a plan? *No.* A new diet in mind? *No.* A strat-egy? *No.* Any reason on earth for my expectation to somehow achieve the impossible and become thin? *Actually… no.*

My entire arsenal against weight consisted of one weapon only: a decision to finish wrestling with overweight in my life and to get thin. *And that, it turned out, was enough.*

One wise decision to finish was all I needed to set up the launch of a lifetime.

One wise decision to finish was all I needed to set up the launch of a lifetime.

Prior to that day, I had dieted. Often. I had dillied and dallied, I had experimented and started. Oh, I knew quite well how to diet. What I didn't know was how to actually *get thin*. I had never properly planned the *finish*.

With military-style authority of a five-star general, I informed my innermost self of my decision to finish. *My wrestling match with overweight is over,* I declared to any stray emotion that might lurk beneath my consciousness, preparing for a sneak attack around midnight. *Bye-bye, extra weight, I'm done with you,* I shouted out from my protected steel cage of shiny, brand-new will that had formed overnight inside me. No more coping, struggling, striving. *This time, I'm in it to win it,* I pronounced.

My 1st wise decision to finish set into motion everything else that followed over the next months. All previous obstacles that had been stacked high and tightly against me soon began to fall, one by one, like dominoes. After my singular decision to finish, everything that later tried to resist me seemed measurably weaker, lesser, smaller than my own fresh, daily supply of irrevocable resolve. No deterrent could stand against my 1st wise decision: to *finish*.

Now I'm thin. Not almost-thin, not nearly-thin, not used-to-be-thin, not soon-to-be-thin, but *thin*. Once the decision to finish was made, *the finish became unstoppable.*

You can turn your back against a lifetime of un-thin living by making a simple, wise, and surprisingly powerful decision: to *finish*.

STARTING AND FINISHING

Finishing is better than starting.
(ECCLESIASTES 7:8)

Starting is fun; it's fantasy, hope, and a reprieve from the unpleasant truth of today. It softens your reality via a mental escape as you visualize change. There's nothing wrong with starting. But if you don't include with it a *parallel decision to finish,* you'll stall fairly close to that oh-so-hopeful starting gate of diet.

Starting commits *only* to *initial* effort. If the decision to finish is absent at the start, from where will rise the energy to *sustain* it? Starting easily lapses into stopping; it's the fast-talking salesman that gets you going. When starting runs out of steam, *finishing* is the smooth closer who steps in and completes the deal.

Finishing changes the dynamic of starting. It captures the wish of your start and cements it into the triumph of your outcome.

Starting has the best of intentions, of course. But starting is moody, changeable and cannot be trusted to sustain itself. Like thin glass, it is fragile and easily shattered. The starter pleads, *I hope it won't be too hard!* Then pessimism sweeps in, whispers discouragement, and it all falls apart. Notice how pessimism knows better than to harass a *finisher?* Because there is no point. It has no effect.

Imagine a long-distance runner nearing the *finish* line at the Summer Olympics. On what is the runner fully focused? She is riveted on one thing only: the *finish* line ahead. Will that runner even *hear* a whisper of discouragement inside her? No. Finishing is like iron. It warns, *Don't dare mess with my finish!*

To say you've started something does not necessarily impress others nor describe you. After all, there are many kinds of starts: a false start, a slow start, a good start, a rough start. But the act of finishing tells everyone *exactly who you are.* That one majestic word says it all: You *finished.*

Starting opens wide the door to future change, and that's a good thing. Starting is pleasant. But have you ever noticed how boring, repetitive, and inefficient it is? What is there to say about the diet you started last year, last month, or last week? The one that didn't work out for you? The diet you haven't started yet? Or the one you plan to start soon, really soon? The act of starting is tiresome and teaches you little.

> *Finishing is a teacher that teaches you why you didn't finish before. It solves part of your life mystery.*

But *finishing…* is interesting. Even thrilling! Finishing slams shut the door on repetitive cycles of overweight. Finishing is a teacher that teaches you why you didn't finish before.

It solves part of your life mystery. In finishing is revealed great wisdom for a great life.

Finishing is like a tornado that lifts every obstacle in its path and hurls it out of the way as it races ahead. The decision to finish sweeps up the debris of your past, along with the clutter of your present, and converts it all into a cyclone that annihilates the extra weight on your body. *Finishing* is pretty awesome.

And you *can finish;* this is one thing you *really can do.*

You *can* manage your appetite, control your impulses, and proceed directly to the finish line called *thin.* Your *finish* may look different from my finish. Your physician will help you define your finish based on a host of factors unique to you, including your age, health, frame, height, and body type. After the great exhale of a well-defined mission, *with the decision to finish,* you will find a way to complete it.

You can achieve deliverance from past diet failures and orchestrate a very livable and pleasing *lifestyle of leanness.* This 1st wise decision will squeeze outside resistance into surrender, including any residue of resistance hiding secretly inside you.

The pull to overweight has been like a cruel dictator ruling your stomach and your life. *And now you're going to overthrow it.*

THE BREAK-THROUGH

Finish. It is the one word that causes future resistance to crumble.

The decision to finish is impenetrable because it has no exit strategy, no off-ramp for any reason. So, by necessity it launches wild creativity within you. It comes on strong to get the job done. *Finishing* has a big, sassy Attitude—with a capital A. It is grand, courageous. *Finishing* thinks like a champion. It needs no convincing. *It thinks you already won.*

It does not waste time pondering *why* or *if*… it only strategizes *how.* Adrenalin rises, awareness intensifies, and a life-size image of your personal finish line fills your whole being. As if looking through a tight lens, you fixate only on your personal bulls-eye, automatically screening out the noise and wasteful conversation of weight loss minutia.

Finishing is highly efficient. *It approaches your challenge by looking back from your finish line.* This singular mindset equips you to cast off future resistance. When your *only allowable option* is to complete your stated mission, there is just no room for needless and time-wasting contemplation. You no longer toy with the enemy called overweight. You annihilate it.

When you make the 1st wise decision to finish, you crush into rubble any opposition to the thin life you deserve. You grow mighty in moments of ambush. Even when the ambusher is a plate of cookies atop the dining table. Especially then.

Not to worry. The will to *finish* delivers a massive explosion of fresh strength and highly focused resolve. It's like a seatbelt that will keep you safely strapped all the way home. It establishes a much-needed boundary between what you need… and what others want.

Finishing is different from coping, handling, or trying again. The will to finish is unfazed by interim twists, unexpected turns, suggestions, moods, feelings or results. Finishing extracts from you a different kind of energy that is creative, convinced, and problem-solving.

The mindset to *finish* is a game-changer that releases you from the stress of the *present.* In the past, maybe you depended on emotional support—which is undependable. Or optimism—which is fleeting. When these ran dry, old habits and well-grooved patterns insidiously returned.

The conviction to *finish* delivers a different future. It pours steel around your will. When every part of your being is fixed on the *finish*, you become a self-renewing source of your own self-support. You no longer need outward praise or quick results to keep you going. You need no one else to make *your* dream happen for you.

> *Finishing approaches your challenge by looking back from your finish line.*

The word finish has breakthrough woven into its very syllables. It hints of deliverance from persistent struggles. It models a very different type of commitment, one based on awe-inspiring mental resolve at a gut and even spiritual level. *The decision to finish changes everything.*

Your Weight: 3 Choices

You have three choices about how to handle your weight dilemma. You can continue to wrestle with it. You can give up completely. Or you can lose the weight for good and *finish* it.

I'm glad I finally made the decision to finish it and I hope you will, too.

If you choose to continue wrestling with it, you'll hop from diet to diet, waiting for one to eventually work for you. Unfortunately, you'll continue to carry more than just the load of your excess weight. *You'll also carry the load of the lifestyle.*

If you choose to abandon your fight, to give up on getting *thin*, maybe you've been fooled into surrender because of the frustration of former weight loss plans. You have a mistaken belief you can't win. You're ready to abandon all thoughts of weight loss and accept for yourself an un-thin life and lifestyle. Maybe you are considering making peace with the excess weight you secretly despise.

Wait! Before you abandon your fight for thin, let's pause for an intervention *right now!* Before you exit a game you mistakenly believe is unwinnable, hear me:

The game is winnable! Come with us. Joy is before you. *Finishing will be the sweet redemption of your frustrating past.*

You *can* do this—and do it *your way.* Before you is a more physically and spiritually beautiful path.

You will finally reset your life in heady alignment with what you believe.

You will *not* be limited to particular foods—or even to a particular diet. You'll *bypass* all these *personal, peripheral* issues and go directly to your powerful core: You'll make 10 Wise Decisions to make and keep you *thin.*

Come on! If your weight is a restraint, holding you back from some aspect of life or interfering against something you hold dear, then it's time to *let it go.* Do it for the one and only body you are granted in this life. You can make a wonderful difference in how well you manage your body—*and how much you get to enjoy it.*

The third choice, of course, is to finish, and that decision is going to change the energy and path of the entire process. Once and for all. Least amount of net effort. Most amount of joy. Best result. Best choice. Finishing is oh-so-smart.

Choose carefully, dear one. For if you don't, an unfortunate choice will be made for you. And you won't like it one bit.

Your life is intended to be about more than weight struggles, starting and stopping diets all the time. It's exhausting to have a constant wrestling match with food. The evil one, *a distractor,* is on a mission to diminish your personal effectiveness through any means possible. It's time to draw a line in the sand and say, *I'm finished. I'm done. I'm in it to win it. I'll design it so that I can live it—joyfully. No more up and down. Not for me. I will finish!*

Without a wholesale embrace to finish, this would be just one more start, with more sorrows, exhausting effort, and defeat ahead. *Aren't you annoyed by this constant clawing of the same old issue?* Think about it for a few days and make a decision to finish it. Once and for all!

Be sure the commitment to *finish* is set *before your start*. Let your entire mindset fixate on your triumphant finish. Let other thoughts fall hazily into the background for now. This is going to be a different head game for you; not one of endurance, but of planning to cross your finish line. Not based on tenuous optimism, but on powerful conviction which will inspire a transformative change in your mental strategy right from the get-go.

After optimism runs its course, it dissolves. After conviction runs its course ... it completes.

Beware: Attempting any weight-loss strategy without the parallel decision to finish is like attempting to start a bonfire with wet twigs. The fire is easily snuffed out.

The conviction to finish is scary-strong. Conviction is a roaring blaze that devours everything thrown into it. Setbacks and obstacles only enflame it.

After optimism runs its course, it *dissolves*. After conviction runs its course ... it *completes*.

Once you've made the decision to finish, at your disposal will appear an untapped storehouse of unyielding might.

From where did it come? You will later marvel.

Why, it came from you, dear one. It came from within you.

MY 1ST WISE DECISION
I Will Finish.

Signature _____ Date _____

Next: Our 2nd Wise Decision will fill your hungry heart and rock your whole world!

I WILL LIVE LIFE LOVED

Learning how to love yourself!

Un-thin people are greatly loved, of course. Except sometimes by themselves. Yet God's instruction is well defined: We are to love others *as we love ourselves.* One of the special names on your own personal love-list is supposed to be … *yours.* He intends a sacred bit of love to be held by you and you alone, to keep for your very own self. *Have you been giving even that away?*

Make a big decision to live life loved.

My husband once made me a loving promise: "You're under my protection from now on." I remember how secure and safe I felt at that moment. Oh, to be under a loved one's protection! Your decision to live life loved is a decision to provide *self-*protection for a special loved one … you. It lovingly puts you *"under your own protection from now on."*

Sadly, we have offered precious little protection to our own bodies against the uninvited onslaught of excess, life-addicting foods that encircle us at every turn. We have not made the commitment to be *"under our own protection."* We don't even know what it means to actually love and be good to ourselves. A mostly unpracticed skill, caring for self doesn't feel natural.

Undefended has been the precious territory of our sacred bodies. We've bowed our good weight intentions to anyone with a stronger will than ours—even while knowing that yielding to them would be harmful, not helpful, to body and soul. No surprise, then, that we, the *overly* considerate, became *over*weight.

Funny, isn't it, how those same, *un*thinking others *un*hesitatingly express *un*helpful opinions? We've been the *polite* ones, *politely* allowing them to overwhelm our personal will. *Protection of self has been absent.* Some of us have so over-learned the art of gentleness and submission that we've forgotten the importance of a well-harnessed will in the earnest pursuit of a great—*and thin*—life.

SELF-LOVE:
WHAT IT IS AND WHAT IT IS NOT

Self-love is an uncomfortable subject. Kind and loving people like us are so afraid of accidentally tipping the love-scale in our own selfish favor; we sometimes go too far in the opposite direction. We give ourselves away to anyone who asks, even though some of those *"anyones"* would be better off without our assistance. We tiptoe around others; *we silence our own personal need for God-ordained self-care.*

Lack of appropriate loving self-care is dangerous to the mind, heart, and spirit. It does nothing to extend our outreach.

Not spiritually, not professionally, not physically, and not socially. Conversely, it *compromises* our effective influence in other people's lives. And, as often as not, lack of loving self-care makes us *overweight*.

Loving yourself is *not* the same as saying, "Me first." It's only saying, "Me too."

> *Loving yourself is not the same as saying, "Me first." It's only saying, "Me too."*

Self-love is *not* a way to edge out or devalue others.

Loving yourself merely adds a seat for you at the table of bounty you willingly serve up to everyone around you on a daily basis.

It adds your own name to that long list of names for whom you diligently care.

There's nothing wrong with serving everybody else first. The trouble occurs when everybody else gets served *except you*. Everybody else—but you.

This all-for-them, none-for-me behavior may *feel* honorable. But it is not. It may *feel* like a generous-hearted instinct, but at its source is a flawed identity that minimizes your own self-worth and exaggerates the importance of others' whims. Living in this relational rut can become a habitual, destructive pattern. Unchecked, it can ruin your life.

Dear one, you are well-meaning, but you've been operating out of false honor. You matter! You were birthed for a cause. Crushing *you* does not somehow elevate others. As a life strategy, this one has got to go.

✤

Maybe you're like me. For most of my life, I waived my personal needs, focusing only on one thing: *output*. I readily maximized care, effort, and time given to others, both personally and professionally. But I minimized the care and time given to myself. Did I consider myself worthy of love? *Yes, I did*. And I thought I loved myself.

So why did I treat myself as if I did not matter, almost as if I did not exist? If that's *love*, then what in the world does *unlove* look like?

I *did* love myself—*as a feeling*. But I didn't know how to love myself *as an action*. As a verb. In order to have any hope of getting thin, I had to make a decision to live life loved.

> *Love was a new action I would take—toward me.*

Love was a new *action* I would take—*toward me*. I would no longer just *feel it*. I would begin to *live it*. This decision changed everything. *It filled me in a way food never did—and never could*. When I felt full from the inside, I needed less from the outside.

⚘

Asking the world to grant me *permission* for the time, space, and energy to care for my very own needs? Foolishness! But I had seriously misunderstood the word "selfish," a trait I had always abhorred. I had gone too far in the opposite direction, even beyond and past selflessness and almost all the way to elimination of self. What I had intended for good (the giving away of *all of me*) eventually became a disgrace to my own self-stewardship. You too?

God has given us this one life and this one body. We are permitted—no, we are *required*, as stewards—to take a little time and care to meet our own needs. Even Jesus sometimes stepped away from the needy crowd in order to restore himself.

(See MATTHEW 14:22–23.) Even he sometimes needed to be alone.

An un-thin person lives like an unloved person. Loving yourself makes possible the self-care to reach a healthy weight.

God did not create us for self-negligence, but for genuine contributions to his kingdom. For that, we'll need a special wholeness from within, to be filled and full deep inside so we actually need very little from outside. We must lovingly protect our bodies from the assault of food.

You can't ask permission in life to be granted the time and space for those things that support, strengthen, and inspire your body and soul. You must simply decide and do. The world will never put your needs above the collective needs of others. If you know and care for a lot of "others," your own turn for self-care will probably never come, unless you claim it. Last on the list? Why, dear one, maybe you haven't made it onto the list at all.

Are you running on empty? Is your tank almost dry? You knew that would eventually happen. You've not given yourself the proper self-care. If you're running on fumes, no wonder you're fuming. If you don't soon begin *the process of restoration*, your irreplaceable inner engine, that marvelous, not-to-be-explained-by-man brand of uniqueness called *"you,"* may burn out. Or implode. Or fade so slowly that no one notices until your light is gone. You may feel close to that already.

If so, worry not. As long as there is breath within you, you can make a wise decision to live life loved. What a grand turnaround that will be! You can reboot your weight and your life. You can quietly start anew. At any age.

And you can expect holy help. Here's why:

The Priceless Gift

Imagine for a moment that you gave a priceless gift to a loved one. It was a work of art designed and created with your own hands. Your prize creation, it was one-of-a-kind, given by you with great love.

Years passed, and you are dismayed to discover your priceless gift has not been cared for at all. Chipped, damaged, unclean, it's been treated carelessly, recklessly, not tended or valued as sacred or special. You naturally expected your treasure would be *treasured*; your prize would be *prized*. That it would be polished, kept whole and safe. But that has not been the case.

Would you be disappointed? Of course. Yet even so, you would long to be invited into the process of restoration of your precious gift. If asked, you would gladly rush in and help restore it to its earlier glory. After all, you created it. *Its condition will always matter to you.*

You are God's one-of-a-kind treasure and *you have worth.* You were artfully designed by a loving God who longs to help restore you. Your body, mind and spirit are his creation, his priceless gifts to you.

Tend them, treasure them, care for them. Do not treat them carelessly or regard them recklessly. Does your life not have great worth? Is your life not a great gift? Will he not gladly rush in and help you restore his gift to its earlier glory?

Carol's Story

It had been a terrible family visit. Everything that could go wrong did go wrong. Feeling isolated and alone, Carol's emotions felt unbearable. And when her world withdrew its safe emotional foundation, she did what she always did. She turned automatically to her "false-love generator," which was food. A poor counterfeit for the love she so wanted, it managed to crank out fake emotional sustenance.

Carol knew in her heart the food would do her no good. But it gave her the momentary illusion of light in her darkness. The food cast a harsh light, an ugly light, but she was too distressed to reckon with reality. *Just intake the food and keep it coming. Fill the emptiness. Get the shovel. It's dark in here.*

The food was a lie, of course. It would not fill up her empty heart. But like a drowning swimmer, grasping in panic for any way to keep head above water, she grabbed onto anything within reach, and she grabbed often. Food was her life raft of choice, a false and mocking "savior." She so hoped it would be her lifeline, knowing all the while it would not.

As Carol's emotional head bobbed under water, her hands clung desperately to life—and the little girl within, that forsaken little girl, remembered food. Back then. Those difficult days of childhood. Not enough of what she really needed.

Funny how food didn't fix it back then, either. It only made things worse. Much worse.

⚘

When you are *hungry of heart*, food is not your lifeline; it's your choke-line. *Here,* taunts the drug-like demon with contorted grimace. *Take a few bites. Here will be ten more minutes of coping.* Then the ten minutes are up, and the emotional edges resume their cruel unraveling. Now what?

Caught in a toxic cycle, Carol had been frantically fighting to regain her emotional equilibrium. She had used food to steady herself, distract herself, medicate herself, save herself.

But when food is used as a dangerous counterfeit for true light, it fills the dark cavern of need … but with the wrong stuff. As medication for a broken heart, food is toxic. Love cannot be found in a bowl. Three Alka Seltzer and three pounds later, Carol felt like a prisoner coming out of a poison stupor.

Oh, Carol! You poor, hungry little girl. It's all right. *You* are all right. It doesn't have to be this way.

When we don't feel loved, every unlovely thing feels like proof.

She only wanted to fill the empty space. But the empty space was not in her stomach. When the hungry part is located in the heart, we must feed the heart. God is very good at that.

When we don't feel loved, every unlovely thing feels like proof

Other nurturing relationships can help, too, *especially the one you have with yourself.*

The years may have taken a toll on the appearance of your body and the strength of your spirit. But God made you—and he loves you still. You are not unloved by God. *And you must no longer live unloved by you.*

Shame has no place in your life of love. Your weight is not the worst thing in the world. There is no weight your body could reach that would cause a perfect parent to stop loving you, or wanting to help you restore your weight to glory.

If your issue is with food, be thankful. For that is fixable, manageable, controllable. Be tender with your weakness and love yourself, just as God loves you. Live in the love of God and in the love of self. Make a wise decision to live life loved.

THE VOICE OF LOVE

As a child, you had many voices in your ear: shepherding you, directing you, limiting you, expanding you, keeping you safe, instructing, scolding, encouraging, guiding. You had teachers and hopefully a mommy and a daddy, perhaps older siblings, maybe a loving aunt or grandma, a coach, a pastor. Whether they were kind or cruel, you were indeed surrounded by leadership.

And then you grew up. You grew past their influence. Now it is your own inner voice that leads, coaches, directs, chastises, and praises you. The voices of your childhood were stilled. *Or were they?*

Have you ever examined the truth, helpfulness, or validity of your own adult *inner voice?* Some of us could use a little help here.

I wonder if we unconsciously adopt the voice of those early influencers from our childhood. I realize I did.

I had unconsciously selected the harshest, most unloving voices of childhood to become my grown-up inner voice. I thought if I could please *that* inner voice, then surely I would be safe and above reproach. My inner voice didn't come exclusively from any one person, but was a composite of the worst, most unloving people who impacted my childhood. If only I could satisfy that mean-spirited *choir* now merged into one painstaking taskmaster-voice that lived inside my head, I would know beyond all doubt that I truly was the wonderful person I so hoped to be.

But there was a teensy problem. I never could please that choir. *There are some voices you cannot please.* If you invite such a mob into your head and permit them unrestrained access to your confidence, you are headed for insurmountable discouragement. *And a weight problem.*

Have you adopted a mean, accusing inner voice from someone in your past? Have you allowed *that voice* to verbally attack without mercy the frightened child within you? Child abuse is a crime, you know. *Even if both abuser and victim are one and the same person.*

Take immediate action, dear one. Silence the inner voice that spits out lies and a *false running commentary* about who you are capable of being, doing, and becoming. Protect that kid within!

Imagine you had been nurtured as a child by voices of love, wisdom, and solid maturity. Voices offering encouragement, strength, and steadfast reassurance. With God's help, *why can't that be your new inner voice?* With a little practice, you can learn to express to yourself kindness, not judgment; caring, not condemnation; encouragement, not dismissal; truth, not mean-spirited lies. Do you long to hear hope? You can learn to *speak* hope *to yourself.*

Is this possible? Even now? Oh yes! Make a life-changing decision today to *live life loved.*

Don't permit suffering at the voice of any bully. Not ever again. *Pinky swear.*

In order to live life loved, you must redefine what it means to be truly good to yourself. In the past, you may have said, "I've had a horrible day. I'm going to be *good to myself.*" And what did that mean? An over-sized, high-fat, high-calorie meal. And maybe you topped it off with a large dessert—the rich, gooey kind that swells the stomach and dulls the senses.

If you want a heavy meal or a big dessert sometimes, then have it. But please don't call it "being good to yourself," because that's a lie. It isn't. Over-stuffing is being unloving and hurtful to you. It's a demonstration of un-love. Real love does no harm.

THE PRICE YOU'VE PAID

You've paid a terrible price for living as if unloved, and you pay it every day. Face it; being un-thin is a lot of work. The energy required to manage the issues of overweight are maddening. They drain you of time, peace, money, space, emotional equilibrium and self-confidence.

Constant eating interrupts your work, play, travel, vacations, and projects. It disrupts your free time, your movies, and your entertainment. Maybe even your sleep.

Eating food eats up your time. It takes *time* to think about, dream about, drive through, prepare, purchase, pick up, cut up, clean up and then to warm, cool, chew, swallow, and digest.

Closet space becomes unmanageable, your hangers and drawers overstuffed with various clothing sizes, yet with very little that actually fits. Lots of shoes, but nothing to wear

> *In order to live life loved, you must redefine what it means to be truly good to yourself.*

with them. You'd buy more clothes, but hesitate to surrender the dream of fitting again into those smaller sizes already hanging in your closet. Anyway, the clothing choices in your large size are limited, and the image they present to the world is *not who you really are.*

Besides, your finances have been drained by the cost of miracle diets, magic supplements, and special plans, shots, pills, doctors, and surgeries.

Self-negotiation accompanies you at every meal. It's exhausting to referee the conflict between what you *want* to eat and what you *think* you should force yourself to eat instead.

Photos are discouraging. In fact, you'd rather *take* the

photo than be *in* the photo. You opt out whenever you can, which only compromises the memories you long to preserve of special occasions, vacations, and visits with loved ones.

You sacrifice many opportunities for fun and adventure, physical activity and romance, sports and hobbies, because it's too much stress on your overstressed body. And swimming with others? *In a bathing suit?* Out of the question.

Unfriendly mirrors ambush you at entrances to stores, ruining a perfectly good mood with an unholy vision of someone *you know you're not.*

Mentally, you're often preoccupied. Then there's the mental fog when the sugar bottoms out of your system. You frequently battle stomach distress of all sorts, including gas, bloating, and acid indigestion.

Intimacy is compromised; you sometimes avoid *touch* to hide *girth.*

You're understandably frustrated and angry at the lack of privacy in which to deal with your weight problem. It rudely announces itself every time you walk into a room, at every encounter with friends—or even strangers, who see nothing wrong with giving you unsolicited advice. For crying out loud, other people have issues too, but they have privacy. Their issues are not sitting on their hips.

And gee thanks, social media. Lately, you feel increasing pressure to look good *all the time*, even to talk with your family on the phone. You yearn for the old days when you could limit your public exposure to one, good, carefully staged Christmas photo each year.

♕

You have paid a steep price for not *living life loved*. What the world sees on your body represents only a distorted version of who you really are.

They have no idea what deliberate exertion it takes for you to be the wonderful person you are. Are you tired? Overscheduled? Overburdened? Over it?

I understand. And I bring very good news.

Your history is not your destiny. Say good-bye to struggle. *This food-pull on your life can and will be broken.* Past diets may have caused your resolve to weaken and esteem to stall. But they indicate absolutely nothing about your ability to overcome. *Overcome you will.*

When you live life loved, you'll birth a new way of life: a confident life, an overcomer's life, a better life than the life you are presently living. You will live in love and prosper in love. The food-grip will release.

Don't get thin in order to be loved. *Get thin because you are already so dearly loved.*

My 2ND Wise Decision

I Will Live Life Loved.

Signature _____ Date _____

Next: Our 3rd Wise Decision reveals and reclaims your stolen thin identity!

I WILL HAVE A THIN IDENTITY

You have a weight identity.
And you can change it.

Ever wonder why your past diets haven't worked for you? Maybe because they directed you to focus on the wrong body part! You were looking for answers in your *stomach*.

But the secret to thin is all in your head.

You do have a weight identity. And you can change it. So, fasten your seat belt. Buckle up. You're about to have an identity change.

You started out thin. We all do. Somewhere along the way, your thin identity was lost. You had no official papers, no weight identity card to validate the weight of the *real* you, so you settled for a most unfortunate switch. Gradually you came to believe a *false* identity about your weight.

Weight identity operates like a navigation system, an

internal GPS guiding you hour by hour to a weight destination. A diet can't take you home to thin, *if thin is not your home.* Diet can give you a good push. But in the end, we all go *home* to whatever weight identity is firmly established in our head. Better find out what yours is!

Around a false, un-thin identity you have made all your decisions about food, at times when you were paying attention *and at times when you were not.* You've been utterly faithful…to a false and accidental identity.

Your overweight identity is false.

But that identity is not truly you. It's all a mistake. A big fat lie about who you are. *Your overweight identity is false.* You have lost your true weight ID. If you've been living this way for a while, you may not even remember who you really are. *Come back to the palace, lost princess. We, the world, are awaiting your return. We need you. Come back home.*

Make a life-changing decision to reclaim your thin identity. This will be a game-changer for you, a tower of truth to brightly illuminate your path on *any diet you choose.* Make a decision of *identity*, not of *strategy*. Strategy comes later. Identity must come first.

Until now, you've made uneasy accommodation for your un-thin identity because you *believed* the lie. It's as if you thought your name was Martha, but your real name was always Marie.

You *thought* overweight was your personal truth—*but it isn't.* You *thought* you had no choice about your weight identity—*but you do.* So let's be done with the foolishness that you can't be a thin person. Of course you can. *You used to be thin!* Don't you remember?

You didn't get to your present weight without first crossing through *thin*. There's not a single instance on the planet of an overweight person who did not at one time weigh their ideal weight, even if it was back in early childhood. You can't have reached *here* without first having crossed *there*.

Make the wise decision to have a thin identity. What a fabulous decision it will be; the easiest path to thin you can imagine. *Your body will race toward thin,* and you will *never* have to *overcome overweight* again.

Like you, I too had a false weight identity. I thought *overweight* was my official weight ID. I tearfully accepted it, tried to make the best of it, and smiled bravely through the worst of it. But once I realized I had been the unwitting victim of a *lost weight identity,* I forcefully shrugged off that old label and began to *act* and *eat* like *the real me*. The real, *thin me*. From identity lost to *identity thin*.

Merging my *outer appearance* with my *inner* identity took a few months, but it was *not* difficult. Even before the *outer* weight came off, the *inner* weight released its grip. I wasted no time with remorse and instead marshalled all my attention on reclaiming what was rightfully mine: *thin*. I wanted it. I deserved it. And I knew it was God's best for me.

Hesitantly, I took my first wobbly steps in my new truth as a thin person. With each day I felt surprisingly more accomplished and skilled, strong and sure. Thrilling is the joy of returning to your original thin identity. How wonderful to know that if you *choose* thin, you *get* thin. Confidence blooms with the empowering fact that *you did the choosing.*

Today, I am at my seventh-grade weight. Can you believe it? Age twelve had been the last time I was thin. My true thin identity, once reclaimed, delivered me faithfully, all these decades later, right back where I belong.

A thin identity is not about changing you.
It's about rediscovering you.

When *thin* is your personal brand and your natural state, you unconsciously begin to design your life around that which keeps *you* being *you.* Those who think of themselves as *thin* make *thin* choices and *remain thin.* If you have a thin identity, you automatically drift toward thin, even when you're not thinking about thin. You maintain *thin* as your normal, natural state of being. Anything *but* thin feels unnatural and strange.

Your thin lifestyle is not based on secret foods or rigid regimens, but simply on you being you.

Your thin lifestyle is not based on secret foods or rigid regimens, but simply on *you* being *you.* It all falls into place naturally.

A thin identity is self-loving, strong and disconnected to careless craving. It seeks above all to protect the sacredness and leanness of the body. It encourages you to eat really well and to enjoy food thoroughly, but it requires food choices to *compete with each other* before one is selected and granted access. Any food not designated by your thin head as helpful or pleasing is brushed aside without afterthought.

FAT HEAD, THIN HEAD

No mere diet has the power to keep your weight off. You knew that, of course. But maybe you didn't know *why*. Now you know it's because you always return to the truth in your head.

If you have a *fat head*—if your mind automatically defaults to *fat thinking*—then you will unconsciously find a way to uphold your higher weight. Think about it; your instinctive food and eating choices have been markedly different from those made by your *thin head* friends. Their choices have kept them thin. Your choices have kept you un-thin.

Be thankful, dear one, that overweight has no power and no authority to attach itself to you *without your consent and agreement*. Food has absolutely no leadership in your life. You choose your weight; it does not get to choose you. You are the leader, food the meek follower. You are the head. Make sure it's a *thin head!*

DIETS

I know what you've heard about diets. I don't believe most of it. I'm not a doctor or therapist, but I did invest more than 400,000 hours having a fat identity—a fat head—before I made the leap to a thin identity—a thin head—so I do have some personal expertise on the subject.

The head chooses what the mouth eats. Your food is chosen not by your stomach, but by your head. On typical days, a fat head defaults to fat-based choices.

Then, when you decide to lose weight, the fat head often chooses an *inappropriate* diet—one that's severely *punishing*.

As if the diet itself could make you become someone you are not. As if it could change your weight identity. It cannot.

Lasting and profound change cannot begin until you make a decision about who you really are. Without a *thin identity*, no diet will work for you. With it, any diet will work for you. Diets are merely passive tools, with no energy source to motivate or inspire, and no power of their own. Batteries are *not* included. All the power is in your head. Make sure you have a *thin head*.

In my *fat head* past, whenever I met someone who had lost weight, I always begged one question: *How did they do it?* What was the secret food to eat—or avoid? Surely there was a magical solution out there. If only I discovered it, I too would finally get thin.

If the person brushed off my investigative reporter-style badgering and made thin seem suspiciously easy, it would only frustrate me. I needed to know their *secret route* to thin, a route that precious few ever discover.

Now I know the secret, and I'm thrilled to share it with you: *It's all in your head.* No diet can accomplish its purpose unless your head is right. Get your head thin and your body will soon follow. It's automatic. It can't help itself. The body always defaults to the leading of the head.

From a *thin head*, you automatically make thin choices—*including* the choice of which diet best suits your tastes, preferences, and lifestyle.

Thank God I no longer rely on self-denial, which didn't work anyway. I now rely on self-identity, which *always* works. My identity became thin. So I became thin. It happens that way.

A *thin identity* gives you many reasons to be thankful. You eat good food for good reason—on your self-loving timetable, not anybody else's. The grip of food releases and you experience food freedom beyond your imagination. You eat deliberately, not reactively. *And you enjoy food a whole lot more.*

FATTITUDES

Wouldn't it be helpful to *know for sure* if your head has been sabotaging your diet? Mine was, and I didn't even know it.

I've created a word, *fattitudes,* to describe my former *fat head attitudes.*

Fattitudes are underlying attitudes that maintain your *fat head* identity. From these *fattitudes* you make all food choices.

> *Once you get rid of your fattitudes, you will get rid of your weight.*

I playfully envision *fattitudes* as burly football player types, whose job is to tackle your thin thoughts. I can visualize *the team nickname FAT* printed across their chest on their uniforms. As the official blockers of thin, the *fattitude* team of negative attitudes will stop you from getting thin by any means possible. It's their job to keep you on the *overweight side of the playing field*—forever. With this team of unrelenting *fattitudes* fighting fiercely in your head, you will never be able to cross the field into the victorious end zone of *thin*. They will block you every time.

But good news! Once you get rid of your fattitudes, *you will get rid of your weight.* So it's worth finding a way.

Here is a sampling of typical *fattitudes,* all of them tall tales and distortions united on their mission to dissuade you. You'll think of many other fattitudes. Make a list; begin to see them for what they are. You're going to have to get rid of them. *All of them.*

- *I have no self-control.* Not true. If you had no self-control, you would be imprisoned. Or institutionalized.

- *It's always been this way.* Not true. You used to be thin. Remember?

- *Dieting is miserable.* Not true. Only *fat head* dieting is miserable because it fights against your *fat head* mindset. *Thin head* dieting is so natural and lovely that technically, it isn't classified as dieting, because you never want it to end. *I did not have one miserable day getting thin. Not one. It was quite pleasurable.*

- *I can't diet.* Not true. You're on a diet right now, today, as you read these words. Whether declared officially or implemented unconsciously, you're on a diet every single day of your life. It may be taking you to a destination other than *thin*, but rest assured, you are on a diet. When you say you can't diet, what you mean is that you can't force yourself to be someone else (*a thin person*). But don't you see? Your original, thin identity was lost. You *are* someone else.

- *I'll never find the right diet.* Not true. Why are you even thinking about diet? Diet is the *smallest* piece of your weight puzzle. First get your *thin head* back. Then the right diet will *show up*, so you can *finish up*. It will be comfortable and livable, graceful and fun, a great match for your lifestyle and personality. Choosing it will be effortless.

- *I don't want to be hungry.* Ahh, you mean you don't want the kind of trembling earthquake hunger that comes at the bottom of the sugar cycle, right? Who would? You've just not yet experienced the blissful contentment of *healthy emptiness.*

- *Dieting is too time-consuming.* Of course it is, the way you've done it before! Who in the world has unlimited time and energy to hyper-focus on thin choices every minute? When led by a *thin head,* your body follows in step. Diet doesn't consume any part of you. It's *fun.*

- *I just don't want to diet today. Maybe tomorrow.* Now there's a royal fattitude for you. First, please get your *thin head* working and then ask yourself that question again. You *do* want to be *you* today. You just don't want to exert the miserable effort to be somebody *else* today. Make the wise decision to have a *thin identity* and then you won't have to officially diet at all. You can just officially be you. Today and every day.

- *One day isn't going to make a difference.* Not true. Each day of life pays compound interest into the future. Today *does* make a difference; it is roaring with opportunity, value-packed with future weight-loss dividends to be paid later. Today is your bridge to tomorrow. Invest wisely in it. *Learn to love today.* Get your *identity* right, and your *today* will be right.

- *Why should I bother during this week after I blew it last weekend, and have a party coming up this weekend, too?* What a fattitude! Thin head people don't think this way. Neither do children. Go to the emergency room right away and ask them to please shrink your *fat head*. Where shall we start?

— *First,* there's no such thing as *I totally blew it.* A thin head doesn't *blow it;* they *live it*—and without the self-accusations, thank you. If you're going to go around attacking yourself, you can't play with us!

— *Second,* a thin head *longs* to balance the heavy food intake of last weekend and the upcoming party this weekend, with some lean eating in between. It just plain feels better!

— *Third,* who said the focus of the upcoming party is *food?* Is it being hosted by rival chefs competing for your vote? I don't think so. That's your out-of-control *fat head* talking. Isn't the purpose of most parties to connect *people with people,* not *people with food*? Thin people will also attend and enjoy that party! Not everybody thinks the party is about food.

• *Holiday season is the worst time to diet.* Not true. Has it ever occurred to you that thin people celebrate the same holidays you do? They manage to enjoy all the holiday goodies in moderation—and stay thin. You can too!

• *I'll only gain it back.* You will *not!*

⚜

How do you remove these disruptive *fattitudes* from the game of thin? *You eject them.* Yes, just like with real football players in an NFL game. This time, you get to be the referee. Your decision is law. Your rulings cannot be overturned. Blow the whistle, make the call, and eject all *fattitudes* from the game.

That simple? *That simple.* Though I have lost 18 pounds off my body, my biggest weight loss is not reflected on the scale. I lost the most weight from my formerly *fat head.* I only wish I could measure it. Fat head? *Not anymore.* Diet head? *No way.* Thin head? *Yes! I'm raising my hand, raising it wildly. That's me!*

STRESS

Do you have stress? I know. So do I. But I'm thin. Thin people have stress, too.

Stress can do many bad things. It can compromise your health, interfere with your digestion, and even make your stomach swell a bit. But there's one thing stress can't do. It can't take you from size 6 to size 16—unless you invite it to do so.

You know those intelligence tests they give to children? The kind with four words on a page, and the child has to point to whichever word doesn't belong with the others? If the first three words are *stress, upset,* and *anxiety,* and the fourth word is *ice cream,* which word does not belong? Isn't the answer obvious?

If the first three words are stress, upset, and anxiety, and the fourth word is ice cream, which word does not belong?

Once you have a *thin head,* stress will be no more a trigger to eat a bowl of ice cream than to wallpaper your guest room.

The *fat head* has made a *twisted connection* between stress and food, and drilled it deep into our consciousness. We have learned to respond on cue. We've rewritten that intelligence test to suit our *fat head*.

When you have a *thin identity*, neither eating ice cream nor wallpapering the guest room seems like a viable antidote for stress. Oh, you might eat a bowl of ice cream one day. And you might even wallpaper your guest room one day. But if you do either, you will do it for *pleasure,* not for phony escapist *"therapy"* from stress. That old *fattitude* lie will have lost its influence over you. A stressful day will no longer bring on stress eating—or stress wallpapering, either.

Eat what you want most, but never—and I mean *never*—eat when you are feeling stress. Never allow a *fat head* connection to reenter your beautiful thin head!

BODY IMAGE

A funny thing happened on the way to the dressing room. The clerk kept insisting I needed a different size from the dress I held in my hand.

No, I explained. *I have lost weight recently. I'll consider myself blessed if I fit into this one.*

Just try, she pleaded.

After her fourth request, I agreed to go through the motions of trying on the ridiculously small, size-four dress. To my amazement, it zipped right up without a problem. I brought the victory dress home and saved it for my birthday, then a month away.

Once I hung it in my closet, I immediately realized the mistake. The clerk had obviously put the wrong dress in the bag. That sleek curve of sheath was cut for a tiny person. No way was the favorite-dress-of-all-time going around *this* body, no matter how thin I might now be. Quick label check. *Wait, it says size four.*

I slipped it on. And zipped it up. There I was, wearing a size-four birthday dress. *It was my first-ever closet dance.*

We who have worn various sizes through the years have no sense of our body size, so we have to *practice* our thin identity. Speak it, live it, wear it. Get used to it! Drill it deep into your psyche. *Your identity is thin!*

PROTECT YOUR THIN IDENTITY

Alice Anderson loves and enjoys her active family life. A fun-loving mom to two teenagers, she has been happily married to Marcus Anderson, her high-school sweetheart, for 20 years.

Born Alice Zimmer, she jokes that her marriage brought her from Z to A. She's a loved and lovely woman. Her identity is strong and secure.

Last year, she endured a tough season of stress due to a situation at her daughter's school. At the peak of stress, she was tired, really tired. On that week, Alice Anderson wrote a check. Startled, she looked down at her signature and began to laugh: *Alice Zimmer.*

Under fatigue and stress, she had for a brief moment forgotten her cherished identity.

Like Alice, you and I may occasionally experience a momentary lapse—of our thin identity. If so, just laugh—then *rush right back to your personal truth* so that a false identity cannot regain a foothold in your life. Your thin identity was once lost. Make sure it never happens again.

I am committed to protecting my thin identity, passionately determined to live my life as the *real* me, not the overweight me

71

I accidentally became when I wasn't paying attention. I was able to finally get thin because my identity is thin. *And yours is, too.* Claim it. Cherish it. Protect it. *Thin is who you really are.*

In the movie *Legally Blonde*, Reese Witherspoon plays Elle, a dippy, blonde sorority queen who wants to get into Harvard Law School so she can win back her boyfriend. After unexpected admission and some early success, Elle experiences a disheartening setback and is ready to call it quits. Then she has an encounter with her mentor, Emmett, played by Owen Wilson. Emmett is a wise, caring attorney who believes in Elle. Frustrated to the point of giving up on her dream, Elle says something like, "I'm tired of trying to be somebody I'm not."

Thin is who you really are.

Emmett responds with my favorite line of the movie. "What if you're trying to be *somebody you are*?"

And so I say to you, dear one: *Thin is who you really are.*

My 3ʀᴅ Wɪsᴇ Dᴇᴄɪsɪᴏɴ

I Will Have a Thin Identity.

Signature _____ Date _____

HOW TO USE A PRAYER JOURNAL

O h, how I recommend you keep a prayer journal! Mine is a *spiritual and emotional mile-marker* and a joyful *source of fresh discovery.*

My prayer journal is a precious record of the most important thoughts and emotions of my life. *Not* a diary, *not* calendar-based or informational, it is filled only with *simple insights from my conversations with God about how I feel and what I sense. Written as letters to him,* it is a breathtaking scattering of thoughts, impulses, prayers, and musings that dot the days of my life.

What an encouragement to re-read an earlier outcry to God and see what he has done! Had I not kept a prayer journal, I would have robbed myself of the memory of many blessings, large and small. I would not have remembered the numerous times God winked at me throughout a process, nor how he inspired me with hints, clues, warnings, and fresh awareness. I smile now when I read those older entries filled with longing, dread, or fear. I laugh to see how he delivered me—above or safely right through the middle of a circumstance.

It was from my prayer journal that I observed and uncovered the real reason I overeat. Only reading it later did I make the connection and comprehend the magnitude of what my very own writing had revealed. From these valuable, God-inspired insights were born the strategy and contents of THIN & BLESSED.

How I love the look and feel of my prayer journal as I hold it affectionately in one hand! With lines widely spaced and a ribbon bookmark, it's a pleasure to write in it for those few precious minutes each day. There is no lock, but since it looks more like a book than a journal, it is easy to mix with other books and tuck discreetly out of sight. One journal lasts four to six months.

For this reason, on the first two pages, I also keep my ever-changing "prayer-list" for all the *special someones* in my life. When your family and friends know that you really do use an actual prayer list, it builds trust. Since this list is recreated with every new prayer journal, you are spared the frustration of a cluttered, non-functional list. I can rewrite my list—*rewrite my heart*—in another four to six months. Some of the prayer-list names are *"lifetimers"*, especially family and a few close friends, and these will be rewritten, *reworded* on every journal. Other names are there for a temporary, sometimes urgent need—or for no reason at all except my love. Special to me are the names of the loved ones of *others*; people I will never meet but for whom I've been entrusted to pray. What an honor! How fun and faith-building to check off an answered prayer with a date and comment

Written as letters to him, it is a breathtaking scattering of thoughts, impulses, prayers, and musings that dot the days of my life.

beside a name on my list. It provides permanent documentation of answered prayer throughout my life. And at times when God's answer was not what I'd hoped, it provides focus to spiritually grow.

The use of a prayer journal is *a most nurturing routine* that takes just five minutes. Remember to write *only* your impressions—*not your activities*—and you don't need to post every day.

Ten Benefits
of A Prayer Journal

1. *It builds your faith.* You see how God moves life's pieces into place to care for you. How just when you reach the end of yourself, he causes change.

   Lord, I give you my attitude. Let me filter life through your lens.

   Lord, I give you my disposition. Let my default emotional state be one of joy (in you), safety (because I trust), and stillness (unmoved by swirling events and an outwardly busy lifestyle).

   Lord, I give you my appetites. You are my portion. You are my food and drink.

   Lord, I give you my talents. Show me your best next step for me.

   Lord, I give you my marriage. Show me how to be, show me what to feel. Show me how to react—or how to look higher still.

   Lord, I give you my family, my friends, my client relationships. Direct my words, my responses.

   Lord, I give you my appearance. May I be God-gorgeous.

2. *It draws you into a more intimate relationship with God,* as you write from your heart to the lover of your soul.

3. *It gives you a tangible witness* and testimony as to the exciting timing of miracles and events. This increases your courage.

   Thank you, Lord, for your kindness to me, your extravagant grace, the answered prayer, and the hope you give to those who love you—the wonderfully unreasonable hope because you are a miracle God. You twist and bend the universe according to your will and pleasure. I exalt you.

4. *It documents your amazing growth.*

5. *It is a safe friend* to you when you are sorrowful. Writing is a wonderful way to *process* and *settle* emotion in privacy. It gives you a much-needed opportunity to vent, to get it all out without risk of making it worse.

   Show me how to love. Again and again.
   Show me how to speak. And how to be silent.
   Show me what is worth my time. And what is not.
   Show me how to be and how to do and how to think and how to be wise. I crave wisdom that will empower me to spend my days wisely and to complete my life with honor and clean accomplishment. Is that okay with you? Please?
   Help me with my family, to love them patiently, generously, and well.

6. *Over time, it helps you see truths about yourself,* as written by your own hand. You will *know yourself better.*

7. *It highlights patterns* that may be useful to you. You'll realize patterns of thought and reaction, patterns of family and friends, and your patterns of coping.

8. *It is nostalgic and sweet,* as are your precious photographs of times past. I was touched recently to find this entry I made long ago.

> *Lord, in Jesus name, help me be the woman you want me to be. Help me accomplish the things you want me to accomplish. Help me know, experience, receive, model, and deliver your love. Teach me your truth, give me your extravagant blessing, and help me be strong, healthy, loved, productive, and full. Help me listen to your voice amidst the din of life. Thank you for every blessing, especially those I may not even realize I have.*

9. *It provides a memory* for your busy mind of the many blessings we tend to forget.

10. *It makes your personal Bible study truly come alive!*

Next: Our 4th Wise Decision will unblock your path to thin!

I WILL FORGET ... AND FORGIVE

Cancel your un-thin past!

M erriam-Webster defines the word *cancel* as to *"destroy the force, effectiveness, or validity"* of and to *"bring to nothingness."* You are going to *cancel* and *bring to nothingness* your un-thin past. *And disconnect it from your future.*

This breakthrough decision comprises two distinct parts. To *forget* is to rid yourself of the bondage of your past—to effectively disconnect the past from the future. To *forgive* is to release the burden keeping you stuck and un-thin.

For this you may well need professional help. Get it. If you need it, please seek a qualified counselor to help escort you through. Dear one, no matter what it takes to *forget* and *forgive,* do it. For it will unblock you. It will please God. *And it will help you get thin.*

I WILL FORGET ...

What if this were the very first time you tried to lose weight? Imagine your body weight, dress size and food intake had been perfect until now. No past programs, no deprivation, no *diet journey*, no gaining it back, no struggle, no issues, no food focus, no rut, no groove, and no path of failure.

Wouldn't there be a blessed lightness about weight loss? Wouldn't it be a quick and uncomplicated subject? Maybe skip a few desserts, eat a little less, move a little more?

Let's get radical. *Let's un-remember overweight.* Make the wise decision to forget your overweight past and start anew.

Part of our weight trap is that we have become disturbingly *comfortable and familiar* with the torturous issues and processes of diet. The cycle of gaining and losing fits us like an ever-constricting glove. Overweight has been unconsciously adopted as part of our identity. It feels real. The struggle feels normal. Perhaps as a survival strategy, we've *made friends* with the captor we mistakenly thought we could not control.

> *Let's get radical. Let's un-remember overweight.*

Well, I say: *Forget your "friend."* What good does it do to remind yourself of all the times diet didn't work? *What is accomplished in your mental recitals of angst and defeat? Forget the words and conversation of overweight. Forget your past diets.* Leave it all behind. Abruptly turn away and never look back. Walk away.

Your history is not like a credit card to which you owe future interest. When you cancel that memory of overweight, *you owe nothing.* It is quite reasonable to make a decision to forget your un-thin history *and sever it from your future.*

Forgetting is part of God's nature, and he has used rather dramatic language to illustrate it: "As far as the east is from the west, so far has he removed our transgressions from us" (PSALM 103:12 NIV).

If forgetting weren't possible, why would it appear in his word?

Turn your *soon-to-be-thin* back on your past—and focus 100% of your attention on your breakthrough future. Remove diet memories from your auto-response system. Delete them from your inner hard drive. *Forget every single diet you've ever tried. Their memory will only weaken you.* Whoever is *reminding* you is *harassing* you. Get a restraining order: no more being reminded of your un-thin past.

I know what you're thinking. *Great idea. But isn't it a bit ... unreasonable?*

Reason is a well-advised attribute. I live my life mostly in reason. But there are times we are better off to *suspend reason.* When you watch a movie, does it heighten your enjoyment to be *reasonable* and remind yourself you are only watching actors read lines? That the climactic scene of good versus evil is reasonably only computer animation? No, sometimes it is more *reasonable* to *suspend reason.*

Suspend the less beautiful part of your overweight past. Cut that cord. Disconnect yesterday's failure from tomorrow's success. Make the powerful and wise decision to forget!

My stubborn weight memories held me bound and gagged and were dragging me to an unchosen future. Yet this did not feel like self-sabotage. It felt like truth, destiny, a natural consequence of my unchangeable past.

Destiny? Nonsense. Those memories were cruelly suppressing God's break-through-possibility that was readily available to me *all along*, and is also available to you—*right now.*

How fatiguing to recall all the diets you've tried. *Forget* your history with weight struggles. *Forget* those un-thin attitudes—those *fattitudes* that have held you captive.

What you remember, you repeat. That's why you can still drive home when you are half-asleep! One benefit of forgetting is that even if you're half-asleep, you won't accidentally drive to the wrong weight destination.

When you remember and reinforce your past lived as an overweight person, you give the enemy a chance to whisper into your head accusing falsehoods about who you really are and what you can *reasonably* expect. And you unconsciously return, as if driving half-asleep, to your distorted destination of un-thin.

Before the next whisper, strengthen your personal truth. You were once thin. Every baby begins life at a very low weight, usually under ten pounds. We grow and we gain, and at some point we stop. You continued beyond your ideal destination. *So what?* Now you are making a profound U-turn to thin.

Thin is not someplace new for you. It is someplace old. Thin is a weight once held by the real you. Is thin unnatural for you? Of course not. Thin *was* you. Thin is quite literally *within* you.

Thin *is* realistic, achievable, and possible for you, yes you, even in your super-busy, complicated, stressed-out life. Thin is natural and comforting. It will feel like coming home, and *the ride home will be a joyful experience.*

Your decision to forget will *not* divert you to a false or unsustainable weight. It will finally unblock your path back to the true you. When you reach thin—and you will—it will not be as an imposter. *Thin is who you really are.* Make the wise decision to forget your overweight past and return to *the real you.*

⚜

Forgetting is so powerful, it neutralizes many moments of indecision. When you feel a food urge, there is no longer a voice to taunt, "That's what you *always* do" or "That's how it *always* is." That evil voice has been erased from your inner hard drive. It is gone.

⚜

As a child, I would comfort myself with frozen toaster waffles. I'd pop in two of them, douse them with butter and syrup, and for about five minutes have myself a sweet bit of comfort. Hunger had nothing to do with it; it was all about the drug-like comfort of sweet syrup in my mouth and simple carbohydrates in my bloodstream. If two waffles didn't sufficiently comfort me, I would toast two more.

As an adult with *(surprise!)* an inappropriate pull toward food, I dismissed any hope of having a thin future by accusing myself again and again of my overeating past. I thought my past—unchangeable and un-erasable—had doomed my chance for *true thin.*

Nonsense!

I say it again: My history is not my destiny. *And neither is yours!*

Is there diet misery in your rearview mirror? Your future is before you! The window to thin is wide open, with a fresh breeze beckoning you. *You can write your weight story any way you want.*

⟐

Forget the former instability of your stomach and appetite. My stomach ruled my life before I learned natural ways to calm my cravings and curb my appetite. After my decision to forget came a *first-time-ever* ability to handle the hunger I always felt before dinner. Astonishing.

Forget how you looked at your worst. Why should I look at photos of my former un-thin appearance? I had a flawed version of normal, but I've been healed. I refuse to attach my personal identity to a higher-than-ideal weight and lifestyle. You'll have a hard time finding any photo of me at my worst weight. If *impolite* others mention it, I do not add to the conversation. There is nothing to discuss. Why? Because I made the decision to forget my overweight past. *It has been forgotten.*

It sometimes perplexes me that small pants fit over my big hips and thighs. But the pants slide on effortlessly. At times my former body image still lingers, but I have made a great decision to forget my former body image and live in my *true* thin identity.

Forget what you cannot do. Maybe what you couldn't do *then*, you can do *now*. I was unable to diet, manage willpower, or fast. My stomach was always an acidic mess. Ulcers were not uncommon for me; my first one was diagnosed at age 14. But after making the decision to forget, I found I *could* do what I thought I *couldn't*. Forget what you *can't* do. You don't yet know the wonder of all that is possible for you.

Forget what you don't like. Never a fan of exercise, I used to repeat the joke that I "never walk when I can sit, and I never sit when I can lie down." My work involves sitting at a desk. Sitting is my normal stance. The last thing I wanted to do on weary evenings or sleepy mornings was drive to some gym where I'd have to mix it up with other people who looked and felt a whole lot better than I did.

But now I've found a different way to exercise, which I like a lot. I'm glad I made the wise decision to forget that I don't like exercise. *Because now I really do.*

Forget what didn't work before. Why remember it? If we had a contest to see who has been on the most diets that didn't work, I would now hap-

> *What did not work, does not matter.*

pily *lose* that contest! *I've made the wise decision to forget what didn't work for me.* Diet memories no longer have the power to hook me. I've removed all traces of those un-solutions from my house and from my mind. *What did not work, does not matter.*

Forget what you did wrong. Forget what you didn't do right. Want to learn from your mistakes? Try the fun process of forensics. With tender warmth and gentle curiosity, you will examine—*once only*—what went wrong. And construct a quick, creative strategy to make it work out better next time. Don't trap yourself into repeating a mistake. Don't stay in that gap. Hop right out! Get back on the joyous road to thin. After forensics, *forget it.*

Forget that you gained it back. Why would you recite such a terrible thing to yourself? Let's not even dignify this by discussing it.

Forget self-confessing defeats. Have you programmed into your precious mind that you "just don't lose" or that "fat sticks to you"? That you "eat a bite and gain a pound"? Good grief! What *other* myriad of defeatist falsehoods have you embraced and made real? Write them all down and stuff them into the shredder.

Forget yummy recipes. In former diet programs, you fantasized about cooking and viewed gorgeous photos of diet recipes you were unlikely to prepare. They only heightened your desire—and worsened your struggle. The diet companies have encouraged us to *focus on* what we should *forget.* Why submit to tantalizing tastes and recipes that extend your time in the kitchen? Aren't we trying to turn away from a food focus? How is that accomplished by savoring new tastes?

Reality check: We all prefer butter to the applesauce substitute and we all return to our favorites in our unguarded cooking hours. So why tempt yourself with exotic diet recipes? Why trigger your taste buds? The concept of focusing on a bunch of new recipes during a weight-loss program seems suspiciously ill-advised to me. Why is it that diet books always seem to include a hefty section of "special" recipes? Add up all the recipes in your stash of diet books. How many of those recipes do you continue to prepare once you go *off* the diet? *Aha.* I thought so. Focus your affection on eating normally in your thin future, and you'll have no spare affection left for all those glossy photos and recipes.

Forget the pain that weight has cost. Remember your wise decision to live life loved? Let that pain go. It serves no purpose to permanently mourn an un-thin past. The past is past. Thankfully you don't have to continue sledging through that worn-out path any longer! Call your qualified counselor. Get all the help you need. We *can* forget pain, even the pain of childbirth.

Oh how I wanted a holy memory loss for my diet mistakes.
But I was trying to forget certain things that I
had not yet forgiven …

I Will Forgive ...

Unforgiveness can make you *un-thin*. What an awful price to pay for an emotion that feels so ... justified. Especially when the person you do not forgive is ... *you.*

Early in my weight loss, after an unfortunate day of high-calorie eating, I wrote in my prayer journal a few short sentences of shocking self-condemnation. Later I stared in disbelief at my cruel words. No wonder I had lived a vicious cycle of overeating and dieting. How could anyone win over such a harsh inner critic armed and ready to smash hope and destroy confidence after every little diet infraction?

Unforgiveness is a matter I thought I had *long ago* overcome. I was deliberate about keeping current in my forgiveness. But there was one person I had somehow overlooked. *I had never forgiven me.*

We, the un-thin, live under a crippling burden of self-accusation, don't we? So habitual is our self-judgment that we don't even notice when it happens. *And it happens all the time.* Every imagined diet "violation" invites self-blame, even if caused by some misfit diet that bears no resemblance to the way we actually live. When things go awry, as they always do, we say very bad things about ourselves—*to* ourselves. It's hard enough that we carry the burden of extra weight. Worse that we also carry the burden of self-condemnation.

Are you stuck in a cycle of self-criticism? I regret that you will remain stuck—and *un-thin*—until you make the wise decision to forgive that beautiful, wounded soul: *you!*

Victoria's Monday

It was a really bad day, the Monday morning after a very tough family weekend that had been filled with negative emotions that swirled like a sandstorm over Victoria's neatly mani-cured life. Feeling emotionally trapped, Victoria had done the same thing she always did in impossible situations: She had overeaten. Oh, nothing impressive enough to be on the news (Suburban Woman Eats Entire Blueberry Pie), but it was sub-stantial enough that she couldn't pretend to hide it from God or from herself.

Victoria had made a significant investment in that spe-cial weekend. In every quantifiable way, she had given her all. When it didn't work out, she automatically turned to her plan B, her robotic replacement for real love. She plugged her gap of sorrow with rich, comforting food.

Oh no, she shuddered the morning after, stomach round and full with excess. *Not again.*

Then followed the usual stream of self-dialogue, the self-accusations, the regret, the sorrow, the feeling of failure, defeat, and hopelessness.

On the brink of depression, she desperately needed a friend.

Then something snapped! Victoria did something she had never done before. Something she had never even considered: She prayed a deep prayer of *self-forgiveness.*

She began to speak to herself with tenderness, love, gentleness and encouragement. And she began to get thin.

And the earth shook. For at the precise moment Victoria forgave her-self for overeating, *she defanged her accuser.* There was an instant loos-ening of the emotional trap that had ensnared her for decades. She then found new space to begin to wiggle out of that trap.

After that life-changing day, she practiced living intention-ally *in a state of loving self-forgiveness.* She began to speak to herself with tenderness, love, gentleness and encouragement. *And she began to get thin.*

Though Victoria would never have acknowledged it, she had been angry, intolerably angry, for a long time. And the person she had been punishing was ... herself! Fury is exhausting—and a key cause of overweight.

⚜

If you've been accusing yourself for a while, you've probably also been keeping a low profile with God. *I so understand.* How can you be expected to pray, no less to hear from God, over the din of angry accusations and defenses going on in your head? We dare not explore reconciliation and relationship with God for fear that to do so might crush whatever little is left of our hope and our heart. Harshly perfectionistic about our human weaknesses, we then distance ourselves from the only one who is truly perfect.

Oh, but wouldn't it be nice to have some spiritual peace and quiet for a change?

If you've done some things wrong *(and who hasn't?)*, it does not mean your entire *life* is wrong. We've exaggerated the implications of human frailty. We dare not admit mistakes, because we fear if we *make* a mistake, our whole *life* is a mistake.

Forgiveness removes self-punishment as a tool in your toolkit.

Condemnation and self-punishment are for people who don't know God. Forgiveness is a biblical concept! Forgiveness of *self* achieves indirect victories you will understand only in retrospect. You'll see!

Make the Wise Decision to forgive yourself! The true

you—the inner you, the one untarnished by mistakes and failures, anger and sorrows—is a precious and remarkable miracle of life. Like every human, you've made an unfortunate choice

Forgiveness removes selfpunishment as a tool in your toolkit.

or two. *Perhaps you've had a rotten start. But you don't have to have a rotten finish. Or an overweight one, either.*

Like Victoria, I had a tendency to automatically switch to plan B in my worst moments. But one fine day, I gave myself a great gift: forgiveness! Ceremoniously, with prayer, tears, and fullness of love, I marked that date in my prayer journal to make it official. A transformational gift it was, with an imaginary gift card that read: "To me, From me."

Now, on the rare occasion of food-regret, my response has completely changed. I am a soothing friend to myself, a genuine ambassador of God's love to the frightened child within me. No longer my own enemy, I am a trusted and gentle advocate. *To me, from me.*

Anyone who has ever dieted has some toxic inner self-talk in their head. *Until you stop shaming yourself, you will never be free.* You are not going to be perfect. But you don't have to be *perfect.* You are *loved.* You really can wrench yourself free—if you will first give *yourself* the love and forgiveness you wish you could receive.

When you make a food-mistake *(and you will)*, learn to be exaggeratedly gentle and loving with yourself, as tender to you as you would be to a little child. *I now talk to myself as if I were in kindergarten!* Very loving, forgiving, full of tenderness. Does it work? *I'm 18 pounds thinner. It works.*

Here is a special entry from my prayer journal just one

month after my ceremony of self-forgiveness. Feel the sweetness and the healing in my heartfelt words to God and myself
that day:

Elizabeth, it is all right.
You are all right.
You cannot be someone else.
But it is worthy and it is safe to be you.
You cannot look like someone else.
But it is lovely and safe to look like you.
I made you and I have stamped you: "Made by God," for
*   my purposes.*
Made on purpose, not to be thrown away.
Treasured by God for all the years of your life.

I invite you to forgive yourself. Please do it today. *How
lovely will be your private ceremony of self-forgiveness in the
sacred presence of God.* Let it out in trusting, broken prayer.
You don't need to read a prayer written by someone else ages
ago. Children don't come to their dad with eloquence. Kids
don't read other kids' words when they speak to their father.

Just state your truths to him—clearly, boldly, factually, *rev-
erently*. Forgive yourself. And dare to ask his forgiveness, too.
God loves you. He always did. Bring tissues ...

⟁

After forgiveness comes grace: authentic grace, not the escapist, hiding-from-truth, I-got-away-with-it variety, but surging,
truth-born liberation. Fresh-scrubbed newness. As an anti-
aging remedy, this one can't be beat. You will be *unhindered*.
And you will begin to rid yourself of extra weight.

FORGIVE OTHERS ...

Let me guess: Somebody contributed to your weight problem. Maybe several somebodies. Or maybe your entire family or work team. *Or your spouse.*

Talk with a qualified counselor or pastor and do what you need to do. But whatever *else* you do, be sure also to *forgive*. Forgive any person, place, or thing that has directly or indirectly contributed to the stress that led you to seek food as relief. This act will release you—and your weight—from the bondage caused by un-forgiveness. *Let it go.*

> *After forgiveness comes grace: authentic grace, not the escapist, hiding-from-truth, I-got-away-with-it variety, but surging, truth-born liberation.*

Let forgiveness sweep like a fresh wave over the whole, miserable history of your weight. Start anew! Forgive those who add to your weight struggle, those who divert and subvert. Let me be crystal clear. I did not say to give in to them. Only to forgive them. You will be *far more able to resist their tactics* (which may even be unintentional), if you possess the relaxed emotional posture of one who is *not* blocked by anger.

You can end the cycle of anger, frustration, guilt, and shame. These are leeches that have kept you far away from thin. Put the self-accuser on notice: *Self-condemnation is over.* No more accusatory whispers. No shame. The enemy has been defanged.

When you shine the light of loving forgiveness on that dark space deep within, you'll soon see thrilling new possibilities—including the possibility to be thin.

Prayer Journal Entry

Thank you, Lord, for ... my weight ... today, for giving me so much grace despite bad behavior. Help me give as much grace to others as you give to me.

⚜

My 4th Wise Decision

I Will Forget. And I Will Forgive.

Especially _____.
(name)

And also _____.
(name)

I also forgive me. And I ask you to forgive me, too.

Signature _____ Date _____

Next: Our 5th Wise Decision will infuse you with more confidence than you ever thought possible!

I WILL FLEX

I have learned to stare down a cookie. Or leave on the plate the last bite of one I chose to eat. My *yes* is *yes* and my *no* is *no*; I am spared the torturous energy of waffling in indecision. And when my answer to the cookie is *yes,* it is a yes of clarity—wholehearted, undefiled and unspoiled by remorse. *What a wonderful way to live. I can't wait to show you how!*

But first, may I introduce you to someone very powerful? I would like you to meet ... *you.*

Get ready, elegant warrior, because the decision to flex is going to change the trajectory of your whole life. Flexing will equip you with *support beams* for your thin identity. No longer tentative, you'll be in control. No longer a weakling, you'll be strong. No longer uncertain, you'll be *confident.* No longer unthin, you are going to *get* and *stay* thin.

WHO'S THE BOSS IN YOUR LIFE?

My former "boss" was pizza, which "paid" me only in pounds. Duped was I into thinking I could not resist the urgent call of pizza every weekend.

Not anymore. I have met my elegant warrior self.

Pizza? Sometimes I *decide* to eat it. Other times, I don't. But one thing is for sure: *I* choose *it.* I make the choice. *It never chooses or rules over me.*

༄

How would you feel if your spouse said, "I want to be faithful to you, but *I just can't resist* the call of so-and-so?" What if your teenager confessed, "I want to be drug-free, but *I just can't resist* the call of drugs?"

Many of us have grown up in every way except in our relationship with food. It's time to put aside helpless, childish ways of thinking about food and eating. Children are ruled for their own protection against foolish choices. *But adults self-rule.* They identify obvious dangers. *They have the grown-up will to resist them.*

> *Eating whatever you crave? That's not personal freedom. That's bondage.*

If you don't self-rule … if you don't develop spiritual and mental muscle *of your very own,* then prepare yourself: something *outside* you is going to rule you. *Let it not be food.* Eating whatever you crave? That's *not* personal freedom. That's bondage. Freedom is being in total control over the actions of your own limbs, not obeying the irresistible call of pizza. You *can learn* to rule yourself. *You can do this.*

Dear one, *take authority* over every morsel you put into your mouth. Don't even whisper weakness! *Don't let anything in this world, seen or unseen, hear you speak of your vulnerability to food.* Why repeat to yourself the weak-willed deception, the lie that you can't resist … anything? Any. Thing. Make the decision to flex your will! You'll see fantastic results very quickly. Flex repeatedly and your will is going to strengthen like steel.

What I Learned at the Gas Station

We all start out with a very strong will. Ask any two-year-old who wants something. Then we grow up—and grow cautious. We begin to realize an ego-driven will can take us all sorts of bad places we dare not go. Misdirected, a strong will can destroy a marriage, unravel parenting, get us fired from a job we love, or generally take us down.

A strong will is safest when restrained. But there are times when we need to *unleash it for our benefit.* Maybe we should learn to think like a two-year-old again. Because sometimes a strong will, *used rightly*, is a godsend. *A strong will can help you get thin.*

A strong will can also save your life. Unleashed appropriately against a foe, it ignites inner resources. Body and mind spring into action when special strength is required in intense situations for a highly focused outcome. Later, you look back and think, *how in the world did I do that?*

Once, while filling my car with gas, I was approached by a disturbing stranger who appeared from nowhere. I felt the hair go up on my neck. I knew his intention was not good. He tentatively stepped toward me, breaking through the immediate area around my car—he was in my space. I had no weapon to protect me. All I had was the gas nozzle. *And my fierce will.*

I narrowed my eyes to pinpoints and flexed every cell of my will to stop him. I would defend me. I would resist him. "Don't take another step," I said quietly, with the tone and inflection of a military general. He seemed surprised, as was I, at my commanding voice. But the will is a very strong force.

He paused in his tracks, uncertain. After a second or two, he cautiously took one more slow-motion step toward me. I removed the gas hose from the car and pointed it at him.

"I. Mean. It," I said slowly, staring hot coals through him.

And believe it or not, he turned and ran away from me!

Why? I believe in part it was because *my will to protect myself was mightier than his intention to harm me.*

That's how it is with a strong will. It can protect you. It can crush opponents *and make them run away from you.*

Perhaps you are like I was before I made the wise decision to flex. Back then, I hadn't known my own strength. Though devoted to self-improvement, both personally and professionally, I had paid no attention to increasing the fitness and strength *of my will.* What a mistake to ignore my body's central navigation system! For it is *in our will* that we make the decisions and take the actions that determine the outcome of our lives.

FLEX YOUR WILL

Let's do some muscle building of a *radically different kind.* Make a decision to flex and strengthen your *will*—the "*you-muscle*" that directs and determines the *outcome* of your efforts. Without the cooperation of *you,* you can do nothing.

It ends today. If you want to be strong, autonomous, powerful, then flex your will.

Every time you flex your will, it grows stronger, thereby weakening by comparison anything that challenges it. If your will has been largely un-flexed recently, then no wonder weight loss has seemed insurmountable! How could it not be? We've believed a life-stunting deception that we are powerless. Oh, the lies we believe. The untruths for which we unwittingly fall.

No longer, dear one. It ends today. If you want to be strong, autonomous, powerful, *then flex your will.* Each time you say no to an urge or impulse, you build muscle... the muscle of your will. This is one muscle that builds quickly.

Why are we so un-flexed? *It's not just you.* Our society is largely unpracticed in the flexing of will. As an option, it doesn't even occur to us. Our language is flavored with phrases that actually *weaken* our will to food, such as *"to die for."* The expression may sound cute, but think about it. Isn't it an insult to you? And to God? Would you really be willing to *die* for a piece of dark chocolate cake?

Has food placed a hook in your nose and a bit in your mouth? Have you thought of food as your master? Have you enlarged its power and denied your own?

Make a wise decision to flex your will.

We make fun of animals that can be caught with food. A mouse loses its life for a piece of cheese. A bear is trapped by sugary food craftily staged in a cage. A fish practically jumps onto the hook for a bite of shrimp bait.

Is that how you want to live? To be someone who can be *had* for a bite of food? Do you want to be the one who is easily lured, trapped and overtaken?

You are not a weakling. You may think your strength is small, but that's only because you've forgotten how to flex your mighty will. *But that's the same will you flexed quite insistently when you were two years old.*

You've unnecessarily minimized your own standard of

control and you've inflated the supposed power of food, mentally magnifying the allure of its bait to your personal happiness.

The out-of-shape will feels like it's comprised of rival gangs in the backstreet, each vying for power. Or as if there is an entire debate club in vocal residence in your head. But when you make the wise decision to flex, the street gets quiet. The mind settles down.

An encouraging thing happens each and every time we make a well flexed food choice: it reinforces that same choice next time. One great thing about muscle: *it has memory.*

Am I perfect in this? Embarrassingly not. But I have flexed my will sufficiently now so that *the muscle of my intention does much of the work for me these days!* Just as when I reach to pick up something heavy and my physical muscles do the work, nowadays my *mental* and *spiritual* muscles are well flexed. They too serve me well. There is no longer any food, *not pizza, not pasta,* that has power over my steel will. I eat them when I *choose* to eat them, when I *set my will* to eat them. *I self-rule.*

Midnight at the Inner Gym

It is midnight. Everyone in the house is in bed, but you're not. You're too tired to sleep. And a little stressed. Dinner has long since been digested and you'd like a little something to … well, to make you feel better. You know, maybe get more relaxed, and maybe more sleepy.

You open the refrigerator. Nothing too exciting there. Then the freezer. And there they are, glowing in splendor … the ice cream pops. The beautifully designed box almost leaps out at you; its very color promising leanness and health! And look! Just 100 calories. That is, 100 calories for one pop. But they are small, so one pop kind of just gets you going, right?

Freeze-frame this moment! *Let's walk through our flex together.*

First, if you eat the ice cream pop tonight, you will be 99% more likely to eat an ice cream pop again tomorrow night. And the night after that. And maybe every night this whole year unless you run out, in which case you will search frantically at midnight for some other even worse choice. You know I am right.

Second, if you eat the ice cream pop tonight, you will reinforce to your body and to your mind that you really are a person who needs a sugar (or fake sugar) pick-me-up every night at about this time. You will train yourself to salivate for the ice cream pop in order to sleep.

Third, a question: If you eat the ice cream pop tonight, do you think it will be *easier* or *harder* to resist the ice cream pop tomorrow night? Let's read the answer aloud together: *It will be harder tomorrow night!* And even harder the night after that. Because you will have practiced weakening your will. If you want to self-rule, tonight is your best bet.

Fourth, if you eat the ice cream pop tonight, you will quite effectively convince yourself that you are a person who simply cannot resist ice cream pops, and are therefore destined to be controlled by their existence. The ice cream pop is your master, and when it calls out to you, you slavishly respond. I suppose you still believe the ridiculous lie that you are weaker than an ice cream pop and therefore have no choice. If an ice cream pop is accessible, you are forced to eat it. Poor you.

Fifth, if you eat the ice cream pop tonight, please know this: it will do you no good. Soon after your carefully well-licked pop stick gets stuffed deep in the trash, discreetly out of view of presently sleeping family members, you will return to your original state of being tired, stressed, and wanting a little something to make you feel better.

In summary, if you choose to eat the ice cream pop tonight, you will effectively practice weakening the muscle of your will. Your poor un-flexed will has been lying dormant within you. *It is patiently awaiting your leadership.*

You want to strengthen your will, not weaken it further, right? So, the singular rationale for the decision of whether or not to eat the ice cream pop is not based upon calories, or whether or not to snack, or about any other *diet* reason you can think of. No! Your steely intention is born of a powerful flex of your will. Because each time you say *no!* to the ice cream pop, you gain the spiritual equivalent of a half hour on the bench press at the gym. What a wonderful, muscle-building workout for you!

So the equation completely changes from a diet-head mentality into one far more compelling than whether or not you can resist the momentary taste of ice cream on your tongue. You'll readily trade an ice cream pop any day in exchange for the laugh-out-loud headiness of knowing that nothing controls you *but you.* It's a bargain trade. You self-rule. Feel it. Power surge! Flex!

THE HAMBURGER GAMES

I sat at the table, mesmerized by the two remaining bites of hamburger on my plate. Not just any hamburger was this masterpiece. It was nine ounces of sirloin perfection, served sizzling from the coals at a fine and expensive steakhouse. I just knew it had been basted with butter. The seasoning was just right, and it was cooked to perfect pinkness. My stomach was full, very full, but I wanted those two last bites.

What was happening inside me?

Like two cowboys just before a gunfight, one of the two sides of my will was about to win. Which would it be? With the drama and impact of an old western, each side grew still. Each drew its weapon of words. The air stopped flowing. I held my breath. It was the moment of the draw.

First up was the whiny spokesperson for my immature, self-centered will. *I hardly ever get to eat a hamburger. I hardly ever get to go to this fine restaurant. I really love this. It was expensive. It tastes so good. It's only protein, for heaven's sake.*

Then I heard the voice of the enlightened me, the surrendered me, the empowered me, the self-ruling, flexing, muscle-woman me, who was aware that I was already happily full and satisfied from a great meal.

Lord, you don't want me to be overfed. It's as simple as that. It's not about diet or about protein. It's about you, Lord. If I flex my spirit-muscle right now, I will be stronger and more powerful next time. I'll feel and be in majestic control of me. That will build my confidence. Lord, I offer these last two bites to you.

And then. The trigger of decision was pulled. Bam!

Which way did it go?

I laid down my fork. The God-side won.

Within seconds of that decision, my spirit soared with a fullness and confidence far more overpowering than any fleeting satisfaction dangled by those last two bites of burger. In fact, the bites were forgotten as soon as the waiter removed the plate.

And then enlightenment flooded my soul:

When I lay down my fork ... I lay down my weakness.

THE PANCAKE DIARIES

I stared at the pancake on the serving platter. Physical muscles still, *I was inwardly flexing my will.*

It was the July 4th holiday and I had made my favorite holiday breakfast: pancakes.

The batter yields six tender, luscious pancakes. I served my husband three and discreetly served myself two. Two large ones, I should point out.

Satisfied after eating my two pancakes, contentment flooded stomach and mind. I was full and happy. Blessed, really. What a treat.

But wait. The third pancake sat there, calling out to me. Did you know that pancakes can talk?

What about me? I'm sitting on the platter and I have to go someplace. You can't reheat me. If you don't eat me now, you'll have to throw me in the trash. Why, that would be a terrible waste and an insult to world hunger. I'm soft, delicious, moist, and wonderful. Don't you want to put me on your plate? Don't you want to feel my texture? After all, I'm just one little pancake. What's the big deal about having a few more bites? Isn't that the more reasonable option? The desirable option? C'mon, I'm getting cold! Hurry!

Has something like this ever happened to you? This is a classic exercise at the inner gym, a great opportunity to flex your mighty will.

How did my exercise go that day?

I took a slow breath.

First, I considered why *not* to eat the last pancake.

I'm really satisfied already.

Therefore, it would be gluttony.

Therefore, that extra pancake would be sin.

Therefore, I would feel regret later.

The pancake was like a double-edged sword: on one side: immature pleasure (which would last ten minutes); on the other side: pain and regret (which would last a lot longer than ten minutes). My pancake happiness would be short-lived and tainted with sorrow. Of this I was certain.

To eat the third pancake, small as it was, would in fact be a way to practice the *weakening* of my will. I would actually be practicing the act of *not* flexing.

That last point is the one that finally got to me. You see, dear one, the decision to eat or not eat a pancake has little to do with the ultimate outcome of weight loss. We've made a big mistaken deal out of small amounts of food, as if a single pancake controls our dress size. Sure, we can talk about the very real concerns of overstuffing a full stomach and of storing the extra pancake as fat. We can calculate the number of minutes we'd need to run on the treadmill to compensate for the added calories. But these issues are *smokescreens* that block the *central truth about flexing:*

A few hundred extra calories mean nothing in the long term of your diet. But the increasing mastery of your will—flexing vs. not flexing—means *everything* to your weight. *And to the outcome of your whole life.*

> *But the increasing mastery of your will—flexing vs. not flexing—means everything to your weight. And to the outcome of your whole life.*

Are you subject to a pancake? Don't be ridiculous. Would you surrender your self-rule … to a pancake? It doesn't even make sense.

Or maybe you are a thrill-seeker, and your mouth just wants *a few more bites of thrill.* Let's consider two pancake scenarios to discover where we can locate the best thrill:

Scenario 1: If you eat the *extra,* beyond-fullness pancake, you will have a momentary thrill of the extra sugar/carb jolt to your system. It will last approximately ten minutes. (I've timed it.) A pancake is like an electrical shock to your system. A quick jolt, quickly gone. Regretfully, that sweet taste leaves no memory in your mouth, only elsewhere on your body.

Scenario 2: If instead you take full advantage of your muscle moment, if you make the quick decision to flex your will against the pancake, if you choose *not* to eat it (acknowledging you've already eaten a generous portion and are completely full and satisfied), then you will also experience a thrill, *a thrill of a different type, one that originates from a different place inside you.* Every bit as thrilling and flood-like as the short-lived sugar/carb thrill, this type of thrill feels flexier, noisier, more like a proud motorcyclist making that unmistakable power-blast noise while charging down the street. It's a flex-thrill, an acceleration of your inner power. The flexing of will produces a thrill that lasts and lasts. About a hundred times longer. It's very real.

Now here's the kicker: What about the *residual effect* of your decision of whether or not to flex your will *or* eat the extra pancake?

If you eat the pancake, the residual is that you'll be over-stuffed, overfed, gluttonous, and overweight. You know it.

If you go to the inner gym to masterfully flex your fabulous will, the residual will be an increasing sense of power that radiates from within and makes you feel deeply satisfied at a gut level with your life and with yourself. Flex moments are muscle moments, and they serve you oh-so-well.

Believe me; your live-in-the-moment stomach will never miss the pancake.

The Spiritual Flex

"Spend your time and energy in the exercise of keeping spiritually fit." (1 Timothy 4:7b)

I take this verse very seriously. Spiritual fitness may not get me into heaven or keep me out, but one thing is for sure: Spiritual fitness makes my earth-ride more palatable and joyful. I don't want my *tomorrow* to be spoiled by my inability to master *today*, so I build *spiritual* muscle. The substance of my days should be about higher pursuits than merely coping. *Especially when on a weight-loss plan.*

> *I don't want my tomorrow to be spoiled by my inability to master today.*

When we are spiritually fit, our *spiritual muscles* do much of the work for us without tiring us. There is nothing stronger than a mighty, God-infused will to effortlessly defend you and your thin body against temptation. So it's well worth getting into shape spiritually. We can do it quickly. And it will serve us well.

⚘

My cousin drove from out of state for a visit. This happens a lot when you live in Florida! I joyfully rushed out to meet her car. Without a thought, I reached into her trunk and pulled out two large suitcases. Effortless for me. Why? Because I've flexed and built new *physical* muscle in my arms. *And my muscles did all the work for me.*

Isn't it the same spiritually? Without spiritual muscles, life seems so hard, even for those who love God. And weight loss? Impossible! Every temptation or obstacle feels like a load we cannot lift. Too much effort!

Not so for those of us who make the wise decision to flex our spiritual muscle. We may not have lesser or lighter loads to lift than those around us, but we only notice the heaviest. When our spiritual muscles are strong, *they do more of the lifting.* Our weight loss plan feels lighter, happier, and less burdened.

None of us will ever be free of carnal temptations. Sins are stacked against us. Our culture is biased against us. That's their problem. *Let's not make it ours.*

We have a choice. We can flex our spiritual muscle. We don't have to be rendered helpless by uncertainty or adversity that would interrupt our weight-loss plans and our lives.

I'd rather practice my flex *sooner,* so I can be more relaxed and free *later,* at those times when my spiritual muscle may be forced into a workout.

But how does one flex spiritual muscle? This question attracts me.

Spiritual flexing is *not* about designating certain foods as bad. And it's certainly *not* about designating *you* as bad! A successful spiritual flex is simply when you execute your will in alignment with what you believe. It's when your words and actions reflect an elegant and fluid agreement with God. Sometimes this takes a whole new mindset.

> *"Do not conform to the pattern of this world, but be transformed by the renewing of your mind. Then you will be able to test and approve what God's will is—his good, pleasing and perfect will."* (ROMANS 12:2 NIV)

Agreeing with God's will is my warm-up for a spiritual workout. An automatic flex.

But if you're like me, you may find there are times you are just not in alignment with God. *Spiritually, I've been lifting the heavy weight of food temptation.* In the *spiritual gym*, weights are lifted each time I choose to forsake gluttony or do what I've said I would do regarding eating. As I've grown stronger, temptations really do seem lighter, because my spiritual muscle is doing more and more of the work.

Essential to all muscle growth is a period of rest between sets and on alternating days. If you, like me, often feel you're getting a whopper of a spiritual workout, you will find spiritual rest to be incredibly renewing.

"Be still, and know that I am God" (Psalm 46:10 niv)

I've been practicing the art of spiritual rest in between vigorous spiritual flexing. Intentionally and trustfully, I try to rest in his love—and his timing. To quiet the anxiety of my perfectionistic heart. And to live more joyfully amidst the din of life.

"Surely, I have composed and quieted my soul..." (Psalm 131:2 nasb).

Wise are we who come willingly to the spiritual gym. *Why, one day, our spiritual muscles will be so strong that for us, life will seem downright easy.*

Your Physical Flex

There is a tired that doesn't go away.
There is a tired you cannot sleep off.
It's the tired of the unflexed.
And it's a life-stealer.

Ahh, you knew we'd get here. Before you form the first word of negative self-talk, I agree with everything you are about to say!

I never liked exercise, either. I was a failure at it, even at school. Gym class was impossible for me, a fervent bookworm. I never could keep up with the other girls, and even on those few occasions when I put forth dazzling extra effort, my reward was usually an embarrassing injury, sometimes involving a stretcher. I had no balance, little grace, and no strength. I got dizzy and nauseated easily. To top it all off, I was overweight and out of shape by eighth grade. Good luck!

As I've grown stronger, temptations really do seem lighter, because my spiritual muscle is doing more and more of the work.

As an adult, my five favorite pastimes all involve sitting. (I like to read, write, think, pray, and cuddle with my husband.)

Did I try exercise after adulthood? Of course I did. About once every decade. But there were too many negatives to overcome.

Gyms were repugnant to me. They looked like New Age singles bars with young, bosomy cocktail-waitress types in sexy athletic clothing. Not a place to make me feel wonderful.

Aerobics had two components I especially detest: speed and loud noise (a.k.a. *"music"*).

Pilates at first seemed a distant possibility until the teacher wanted me to move in a way that made my kneecaps almost come off.

The one and only thing that did seem possible was walking on a treadmill. I was thankful to have one in my own home, which I did use, on and off, for years. But I wasn't fit. And I wasn't thin.

For those of us blessed with the ability to move, physical flexing is crucial, for more reasons than we have considered.

We already know that without it, our health and quality of life are sorely compromised. Without added muscle mass generated by flexing, we have to eat pitifully little in order to get and stay minimally thin.

Flexing supports posture, grace, strength, digestion, elimination, mood, stress relief, bones, vitality, appearance, confidence, and anti-aging efforts, to name just a few of many benefits.

But there is something else. Without physical flexing, *the impact of our lives* may well be at risk. I want my life to have impact, and I know you do, too. Paul of Tarsus, a spiritual giant who wrote much of the New Testament, expressed concern that if he didn't *discipline and master his body* after preaching to others, he might himself be disqualified. (See 1 Corinthians 9:27 Phillips.)

But what to do when not one single exercise alternative seems inviting—or even possible?

I was without answers. I prayed to find my personal *yes*. I yearned to discover even one exercise I would not detest and that I might actually be able to perform. I opened myself to unknown exercise alternatives and submitted myself to the Holy Spirit's leading and opportunity. Deliverance came via an unexpected and non-threatening side door.

I met with a surgeon about my painful, troublesome knee. Surprised and grateful that he recommended physical therapy over surgery, I was willing to give it my all for twelve weeks. Little could I have known what was ahead.

God used the words of a physical therapist to change my life. Kind, calm, and systematic, her gentle unimposing logic was impossible to resist. Her words stung me, at last piercing my immature, lifelong resistance to exercise. Here's what she said:

"People come in with an injury and just want me to fix, heal, or strengthen that one body part. You want me to fix your knee. But nothing about the body is "one part." Everything is connected. No part works alone. To fix your knee, we have to strengthen other body parts that your knee depends on for support. We have to build the muscles around your knee, and not just on your legs, but also the muscles on your hips, stomach, and even on your rear. We have to increase your stability and balance, too.

"If we don't do all these things, then there is little relief I can offer you, and it won't last. Without building supportive muscle, along with balance and stability to help your knees do their job, you will never have the mobility and pain-free life you want."

She paused, expecting no answer. The ball was in my court. This time, for the first time, I decided to grab that ball and run with it. God had answered my prayer by giving me a new chance *and* a new will to say yes to exercise. I knew the rest would come soon—and it did.

PRAYER JOURNAL ENTRY

Lord, I looked at my fitness calendar. I stand in awe, in wonder, in appreciation—at how you work the timing of events. At how you wink at those who love you.

My physical therapy was administered at a local hospital attached to a fitness center: a gym. But this gym was very different from those I had seen advertised. This one was filled with normal people who were above a certain age and exhibited below-normal fitness levels. Everybody wore regular, non-trendy clothes. My kind of people!

It was a quiet place; soft colors, no music. I saw lots of staff with medical name tags guiding lovely, imperfect people, many of whom were obviously recovering from injury or trauma. I felt safe there. I felt an affinity there. As a hospital facility, the fees were tiny and required only month-to-month membership.

The first instructions I received were "no treadmill." *I tried to feign disappointment!* After a month, I was instructed to walk on the treadmill for two minutes. Two blessed minutes. I twinkled with the authority of my professional excuse. *"Hey, nothing I can do about it,"* I explained to my athlete-husband. "I'm only *allowed* to do two minutes."

I soon witnessed up close the astonishing power of setting *tiny goals.* It hadn't even occurred to me to mentally resist something I could complete in the space of a television commercial. Though it probably took more than two minutes just to lace up my shoes, at the end of each two-minute treadmill "workout," *I had completed a goal.* I had finished something. I had achieved a victory.

Gradually as my knee improved, I was brought up to five treadmill minutes, then ten. A new affection was forming. I was beginning to associate the treadmill with happiness and success. After all, I was racking up so many "wins," albeit in two to five-minute increments.

Eventually I expanded to twenty minutes *(easy),* and one day I surprised my physical therapist (and myself) by walking thirty minutes. *What a little show-off!* By then it just felt natural, good, and right. Then unexpectedly, the ante was upped.

I was instructed to add a steep incline for five minutes in the middle of the workout. I tried it, and for the first time ever, I broke a sweat. But by then, that, too, felt just fine. *Better than fine. Exhilarating.*

And now? Why, I do at least forty-five minutes on the treadmill without thinking, including several bursts of a nearly vertical incline. I can do this when half asleep—and I have. My energy has soared. There is no resistance in me whatsoever. Wonder of wonders, *I actually enjoy it.*

I've learned a big secret: that the littlest moves can pay the biggest dividends. Some of my little exercises would appear to an observer to be nothing. A foot moves a few inches. A hip lifts and drops a few times. But flexing produces amazing long-term changes.

In the past, I was always tired. I think I was born tired. *But not anymore.* My posture had slumped since middle-school. I had no endurance. I was weak. I had no balance. I had no physical self-confidence. *But not anymore.* Regular physical exercise has changed *everything.*

Exercise is one way I give *love* to myself. And through it, I acknowledge God's love for me. It's how I honor his gift of a functioning body, something *not everybody* has been given. I offer the Lord exercise as my thank-offering for a body that is able to move. Yes, I consider physical exercise as part of my worship, part of my stewardship of the gifts he has given me: the extravagant gifts of life and limbs, freedom and opportunity.

As my twelve weeks drew to a close, my physical therapist urged me to continue strengthening my knees *on my own* for four months, after which we would do a second series of physical therapy.

On my own? I don't think so.

I tentatively set an appointment with a personal trainer. This was an expense to be carefully considered. But after honestly analyzing my former cash outflows, some reprioritizing of spending was clearly in order. Premium ice cream, I admitted to myself, had not exactly been free.

When I was introduced to the personal trainer who had been deemed the best fit for me, I gazed in awe. She was beautiful. So truly fit, graceful, and strong.

And here was my hope: She was my age—and dear one, I am reeking with maturity. *That's* when I knew this fitness opportunity was for real. Yes, it would be possible. Even for me. *Even for you.*

Initially, the only reason I was faithful to my appointments was to avoid paying the cancellation fee. But once I was there, it was fun. It felt good. Gradually, going to the gym became my new normal.

Your decision to flex physical muscles is intended to add strength and joy into your body, not to be a punishment. Therefore, the *experience* should be designed to be as fun and stress-free as possible. Never did I force myself to do a single thing that differed from my preferred style and preferences.

First, I just agreed to show up. That, in itself, was a triumph.

First, I just agreed to show up. That, in itself, was a triumph. Then, at the gentlest pace and in the smallest of ways, I stretched myself. And did it consistently. I showed up again and again. I started by lifting two-pound rubberized weights in children's colors. I would unabashedly high-five myself in dramatic congratulation for just getting through a half-hour with them.

As the weeks became months, I found myself no longer

resisting any part of my workout. Then looking forward to it. Then craving it! I was beginning to feel something I'd never felt: muscles! New, lovely little muscle bumps were beginning to appear on my arms and legs.

Most fascinating to me were the anti-aging effects of flexing. These were a big, unexpected blessing. My posture, which had always been awful, improved radically as I developed the back and core strength to finally stand upright. This alone took years off my appearance. I had tended to move slowly and a little too carefully, but became one who springs into action with pep. Stunningly improved were my balance and stability, a core component of anti-aging. Though I do not do yoga, I do now stretch. The littlest amount of effort done consistently for modest periods is what made all the difference for me.

Best of all, *my weight started coming off more rapidly in my fourth month than it had even in the first weeks of my 10 Wise Decisions.* Weight loss accelerated when I began to flex my body.

How might you choose a trainer, fitness class, or gym?

If you can find a fitness center connected to a hospital, I'd try that first. They are often non-profit entities whose commitment to wellness is stronger than their commitment to profit. Their focus seems more about health and less about frivolity. I've also heard great things about some local YMCA or community gyms.

I urge you to set *tiny* but *regular* habits, routines, and goals. *Tiny goals.* Not large. I know this is opposite of what you've heard before. But then, what you've heard before has not worked very well for you, has it?

No exercise self-talk! Mute the inner voice on this one. Refuse to engage in *any* conversation with self about *"how you feel"* about exercise or whether you should show up for your appoint- ments! Some things you don't ponder, you just do. When you go to your bathroom sink in the morn- ing, do you first ask yourself how you *emotionally feel* about brushing your

I don't care how I feel about exercising. I don't need to know!

teeth that day? No. You just pick up your toothbrush and do what you have to do.

I don't care how I *feel* about exercising. *I don't need to know!* I don't permit any negative part of me to have a voice or a vote. In fact, I have a zero-tolerance policy for *inner exercise negativity.* I have flexed my will to flex my body, and my emo- tions have learned the drill: *Vote for health—or you won't get to vote at all.*

If there is any way for you to exercise *early in the day,* I rec- ommend it. For those of us who tend to put everyone else first, days can be easily derailed. Let other aspects of your day get derailed if they must—*but not this healthful part.* This is your body. Not a car. You can't trade in your body—not tomorrow, not in twenty years, not ever.

Think of it this way: Picture two cars. *Both were built in the year you were born.* One was recently auctioned in gleam- ing splendor to a wealthy devotee who paid an eye-popping price. The other car was long ago sold for scrap. What do you suppose is the single biggest difference between those two cars of the same make, model and year? Only one thing. *Mainte- nance.* It's all about the maintenance!

If you exercise with a personal trainer, their time is not

cheap, so use it wisely. Work with someone you trust and respect: a qualified professional. This is an expensive professional relationship. Conversation should be about fitness, nothing more, with their professional attentiveness on you throughout the session. They must focus on you, grow you within your comfort zone, be safety conscious, and provide genuine coaching and encouragement.

Don't sign for any long-term commitments at a gym. In entering such a contract, we hope the financial commitment will make us show up. After a few weeks, it won't. Unfortunately, financial commitment has no lasting power to motivate us. Gyms know that, of course, and exploit it for profit.

Rather than pushing yourself *against* your natural exercise preferences, *try to identify what they are.* Be clear, intentional, and specific. You really can find ways to increase fitness *within your own style.* For me that means serene colors, quiet atmosphere, and no fast or jerky movements.

You may love to exercise in a community of friends, with stimulating music. Know who you are. If you are extroverted, sample every kind of group exercise class known to man and try every single variety until you find one you actually look forward to.

Before you move a muscle, check with your doctor! I did, complete with a full-panel blood test. This assured both doctor and patient that there was nothing wrong with me—except that I was unfit.

No all-or-nothing attitude. That's for sissies, which is not you. Gently grow your beautiful future muscles into what they might be. Be who you are, but be the best you can be. I still don't exercise daily or when traveling. I wish I did. Maybe that will change one day. But I now exercise at least three times per week, and for me that is a stunning and thrilling achievement worthy of the highest celebration.

CARDIO-LESS

I've never liked to jump around. It makes me dizzy. Add loud music and I get a headache. I was willing to change, to be open to a new outlook. Thankfully, it was not necessary.

I'm told our heart valves need to be pumped with intensity to increase fitness. But how to create *fun* out of dreaded cardio? Well, I found a way: H-G-T-V. I only get on a treadmill if I can time it to watch one of my favorite decorating shows! The show is what gets me on and *keeps me on* for the full prescribed time period, because there is no chance I'll willingly miss the final moment of the show's "big reveal."

☙

At this point, the gym is an integral part of my life and brings me much happiness. My fit husband teases that I am a "gym rat," which delights me because we both know that clearly I am not. Will I ever be like those athletes or blonde bombshells on television? Not in this lifetime! But I am soaring with pleasure over the woman I am becoming: physically strong, fit, and confident.

If I, with my baggage of anti-exercise idiosyncrasies, have managed to find fitness happiness, then surely you can, too. This can be you. *This should be you.* You deserve it at least as much as I do.

Let your 10 Wise Decisions lovingly surround you. It's worth whatever time it takes for you to figure this out, because flexing is a crucial link in your quest for healthy thin.

Create a *routine* out of it. Make a *game* out of it.

Decide that it's typical for *thin women like you* to exercise.
Forgive yourself for not exercising in the past.
Forsake any hint of former resistance.
Reconsider exercise as a way for you to *live life loved.*
Forge a personal new path to fitness.

You can do this. And to live the beautiful life you want, *you must.*

Self-rule is the ultimate confidence generator; its glow and glory radiate from the face and elegant demeanor of one who has mastered *self.* Wise and wonderful is the decision to flex your body, mind, and spirit!

My 5ᵀʜ Wise Decision
I Will Flex.

Signature _____ Date _____

Next: Our 6th Wise Decision will reveal and annihilate a hidden cause of overweight!

I WILL FORSAKE

The inexplicable joy of less.

T he fire of my passion for thin was stoked by my Christianity. I love God. I wanted him to fix what was wrong with me.

For me, the time was coming to dethrone the false gods of appetite and craving, which held a merciless grip over my stomach, my thoughts, and my time. For too long had I coped with these deceitful gods in much the way one resigns to a minor ailment that is ever present, never to be cured, only somehow managed with the least strain and distraction one can orchestrate on any given day.

I made a wise decision to forsake food sins.

I knew there was more to our diet struggle than just our childhood or our habits. For many of us—though we didn't know it, didn't intend it, never meant it to be—that root cause is sin. Darkness doesn't just happen at night. There is darkness around us and there are false food-gods we may unknowingly be serving. *"Those who worship false gods turn their backs on all God's mercies."* (JONAH 2:8 NLT)

When we joyfully forsake false gods that have ensnared and locked us into a weight struggle, *new mercies await*. Weight loss becomes far easier than we would dare to imagine.

Freedom is just one decision away from you right now.

Funny how I had unknowingly shut God out of this central part of my life. *Lord, I give you myself—but not that part.* A person of faith, I had long considered myself *"sold out to Christ."* But I was *sold out* to pizza, really, or to whatever smelled good to my ever-needy stomach. I had artfully created a disconnect between *my* eating and *his* Lordship. Oh, how I had *sold myself* short.

Why do man-made diets never seem to work? Because the world's food and diet wisdom, though helpful, does not overcome sin. The *diet du jour* tries to stand on its own, as if it contained some innate power. But God's wisdom is not exchangeable for any other. Every worldly replacement for truth is a salute to un-truth. Oh, dear one, we've been expecting God to bless something he's never been a part of: our food intake. We've asked the Holy Spirit to infuse mighty power from on high to a private, self-indulging space within us where he has never been granted entrance. *Where other gods rule.*

In our heart of hearts, we know the craving stomach is a dark place of want and grasping. It's a shadowy place where truth and freedom are *smothered under the false god of excess food*. A frightening place with no light, the craving stomach is where we go to feel better. We tell ourselves we go to God, *but we really go there*. God is the God of most of our life, but there is a different god being served there: *the merciless god of unrestrained appetite*.

Our Holy Father is not Lord of that space. His law is not served. His principles are not applied. And his blessings upon our weight-loss schemes have been noticeably absent.

God created us, loves us, and yearns to be invited into every inner space, including the darkest of darkrooms. His dazzling light wants to shine—even there.

So what would you guess happened when he was finally granted tearful, tentative access to my untamed appetite? Total transformation. Believe it, dear one. I've lived it.

There is nothing like the power of God to break through an impasse, stimulate change, and deliver us, body and soul, into a preferred future. A preferred *thin* future.

Make a wise decision to end the influence of this false god. Shake off the sin-shackle so that while eating well, you may also live your life—*your authentic, thin life*—without unproductive distraction and needless serve-no-purpose heartache.

GIGL

What would cause a follower of Christ to overeat? It's a reasonable question. Why do we seek more, want more, ask for more, and consume more than is normal to healthfully sustain us? I wanted to know why. *Because I did it.*

The question bugged me, nudged me. Deep down, I knew the extra weight I dragged around, though small, was bondage. I was its slave. There was no way to soften that truth.

> *What would cause a follower of Christ to overeat? I wanted to know why.*

My extra weight didn't make me a bad person. It didn't render me useless to God or to others. It wasn't a capital offense. Its impact on my life was manageable—and all too familiar.

Perhaps your extra weight is no problem to you. Maybe you alternate between ardent passion for food and your annoyance at its consequence on your body. If so, you have my empathy and my respect. I've been there, brother. I get it, sister. *Your overweight does not offend me.*

But think it through. Why would we eat past health? Past hunger? *Past reason?*

I believe there are four spiritual reasons. Four false gods of food that I've journaled about for a long time, using a secret code: GIGL (giggle). I've used the acronym covertly for many years, fearing that if others discovered what GIGL really meant, they might think poorly of me. *As if they hadn't noticed my hips.*

GIGL stands for the four food-gods: Gluttony, Idolatry, Greed and Lust. And there it is. My secret's out!

I don't want GIGL in my life. Partly because of who I am, *and mostly because who God is.*

I Will Forsake Gluttony

Near the end of a lifetime filled with self-indulgence, King Solomon said something interesting: "No matter how much we see, we are never satisfied; no matter how much we hear, we are not content." (ECCLESIASTES 1:8)

What is gluttony? It is eating more than we need for satiety. Indulging in more food than our stomach needs or wants. It is intentionally overeating past a full stomach.

Why would someone who loves God knowingly eat to excess? I sometimes did—and am still sometimes tempted. But things are different now. I no longer want repentance to be my theme song for food. I don't want *any* foods, especially those I love most, to be *tainted* by gluttony.

Beyond sin, overeating is a cycle of abuse. Self-abuse. *Not for me. Not anymore.*

What is the end-game of giving in to the cycle of appetite, craving, lust for food, and endless snacking? Will enough ever be enough? When will it end? And what is its reward?

Most of my friends happen to be thin, which has allowed for more than a little up-close study. Dining with them on countless occasions, I've watched with fascination as they chose fried chicken, apple pie with ice cream, and all manner of diet no-no's. But one thing I've never seen them do is overeat. *Not one thin friend. Not one time.* Thin people are not gluttonous. They eat very well, but they do not over-stuff themselves. To watch them dine is to watch rightness, loveliness. I love to watch.

Gluttony is such an awful word; we do not use it in polite society. But we must at least acknowledge it *privately* if we are ever to make a decision against it.

Gluttony can insidiously infiltrate even a person who is careful with diet. It doesn't just show up on Thanksgiving Day. It may beckon as you sit down to a monstrously sized salad that masks from your consciousness a desire to stuff yourself full. Gluttony is *not* about sinful *food*. It is about a sinful *state of mind*.

> *Gluttony is not about sinful food. It is about a sinful state of mind.*

An interesting thing about gluttony is that we can't and don't measure it. After eating gluttonously, we rush to the scale to see the weight we have gained. But we don't measure the sin of gluttony that *causes* gain.

Though it is hidden from the scale, gluttony is easily observed by others. I don't want to be the person whose calling card proclaims, "She is the one who is overfed." Not me. I want to enjoy all food with moderation and restraint, including salads. I want one true God in my life and no other gods. *I will push the excess away.*

Gluttony is one of the seven deadly sins. Aside from what it does to the body, the greater damage is done to the spirit, which becomes dangerously dulled. *I'm afraid of that dullness. I don't want it in my life, and believe me, neither do you.*

I made the wise decision to forsake gluttony, to eat wisely and with godly restraint. To enjoy food moderately, circumspectly. To make food *less* about food, and more about rightness with him. To consider eating an act of praise, *and stopping an act of worship.*

I Will Forsake Gluttony.

Signature _____ Date _____

☙

I WILL FORSAKE IDOLATRY

When we use *food* to do God's job, it is idolatry. It intentionally bypasses prayer and goes directly to food, ignoring God's explicit instruction that we are to come only to *him* for what we need. Idolatry is *when we turn to food instead of to God* for our comfort, relief, help, aid, love, safety, loneliness or emotional support.

Our godless society finds that adorable! It is considered *cute* to crunch, chew, or sip when we are angry or upset. Movies show the adorable heroine eating a pint of ice cream right out of the container after she breaks up with Mr. Right.

We trivialize idolatry at our own peril. We have deluded

ourselves. Food can never give us any *real* help at all. Food won't fix it.

Idolatry is a grave sin—and it's a biggie. We are to turn *to God alone* in our anger and our despair, *to God alone* for our comfort. *To God and not to any other thing.* Anything *else* we turn to *instead of* God is a *false* god.

I thought it was just my own faulty wiring that had caused me to turn to food at moments of distress, I did not comprehend that I was *committing idolatry.*

Idolatry is sin. Until I was willing to forsake it, I could not please God or *receive his mercy over my weight struggle.* And I could not get thin. When I did forsake idolatry, I easily slid down to thin.

Idolatry hides out in some very sweet people who yearn only to survive another moment of pain and who sometimes forget in moments of despair to *pray*—instead of eat.

There is a better way to live. Have you ever noticed that naturally thin people don't process stress by eating? Stress doesn't trigger an urge for them to *eat something right now* in order to survive another minute of their pain.

If distress is in your heart and you find food in your hand, ask, *Lord, is this thing that I hold in my hand, a lie?*

"Whenever you have thrown away your idols, I have shown you my power." (ISAIAH 43:12)

I Will Forsake Idolatry.

Signature .... Date ....

✧

I Will Forsake Greed

Greed is excessive, extreme, selfish desire; wanting more than our share. It is thinking about a second portion even before we finish our plate. Greed is hoping the other family members will want less of the cherry pie, so we can eat more.

Do we all have greed? When did we get it? How can we overcome it?

Kindergarten. Mrs. Salisbury's class. I have an unfortunate mental video of what I, the five-year-old, asked and what she, the good teacher, answered.

The class was having a special treat: peanut butter and jelly half-sandwiches. I don't recall being offered snacks in the classroom. At the time, it seemed a very big deal.

I had never before put grape jelly on peanut butter, and the first bite sent a sugar thrill through my five-year-old blood-stream. I gobbled down the rest of my half-sandwich quickly. And then I said it. The words I still wish I could take back, more than fifty years later: *May I have another half, please?*

Kind Mrs. Salisbury looked down at me with reproach. *You've already been served. Others have not. You may not have more until all the others have been served.*

There it was. *Shame.* She nailed me. Why did I ask for more? I was certainly not an under-privileged child. But greed had reared its grasping head when I was only in kindergarten, before I could name it, understand it, or spell it.

Then there was that butter cracker incident, when only two remained in the box and my brother was younger—and slower than me. Oh my! Greed is very unattractive.

The temptation to greed is unpleasant to think about, difficult to write about, but *foolish to ignore.*

If you find yourself eating because of an inner pull *not directly caused by hunger,* a pull you do not understand, then do something dramatic that will get the attention of heaven and hell: Stand up, walk to the trash, and with great drama, make a statement of faith, something like, *I love you, Jesus, far more than food!* And throw the last bites into the trash.

What a fearsome demonstration of strength and will. It makes a statement that reverberates in the deepest recesses of spirit. I've done this with the most treasured of foods, and it sends a shock to the inner self that one does not soon forget.

It *destabilizes* inner greed, while surging a thrilling power through your spirit. *You cannot imagine the raw confidence that arises from such an act.* Talk about *giggling!*

I am on guard against the false god of greed that seeks place or power in my life. To remind greed that it has been ejected from my life, I always place myself near the *end* of any food or buffet line. *The very act makes me smile.*

I Will Forsake Greed.

Signature _____ Date _____

☙

I WILL FORSAKE LUST

"Above all else, guard your affections." (PROVERBS 4:23)

Lust isn't just about *that.* It is also the longing and fantasy for *food.* It's having an inappropriate food desire that crosses the line from mild anticipation to sin-like passion. It's when food preoccupies your mind, fills your fantasy life, and swoons your heart.

Our society considers food-lust an appropriate affection, a hobby, a cultural norm. We even have pleasant-sounding names that make it seem acceptable and interesting: *foodies, gourmands, and other socially accepted nicknames.*

I don't want to be a foodie. I don't think the sin of lust is a very good idea, no matter what cute name you give it.

Lust for food is a false god that consumes mind, heart, and spirit as we plan for it, attend to it, save pictures of it, pay homage to it, watch television shows about it, and even dream about it. Media and magazines that cater to *foodies* are big business.

Even a commercial diet program or plan can generate lust, if it over-focuses on food. Isn't that the flipside of the same coin? Aren't we to turn *away* from food, not just refocus our affection *from another angle?*

I try to imagine how God feels about the false god of food-lust. He says in his word that he is a jealous God. (SEE EXODUS 20:5 NLT)

I wonder if we can understand how he feels. If our spouse glances attentively at someone of the opposite sex, we feel annoyed, even angry. Similarly, when we lust after food, then in God's eyes, we too are "glancing attentively" at the wrong thing. Our Father doesn't like it one bit.

I used to have too much *enthusiasm* for food. Now I'm careful to guard my affection, my attention, *and even my words. For me,* it is not a good idea to watch cooking shows or pore over glossy photos in cookbooks. I have *tempered my language* and my *descriptive words* from extremes like *adore* and *love* to milder terms such as *like* and *nice*. I now say the entrée tastes *good*. Period.

And when eating, I am watchful for more than just calories. Where there is passion, there is potential for food lust. I want no part of it.

Make a wise decision to forsake the food-sins that so easily ensnare. Forsake GIGL: *gluttony, idolatry, greed,* and *lust.*

My 6ᵀᴴ Wise Decision
I Will Forsake Lust.

Signature _____ Date _____

Next: Our 7ᵗʰ Wise Decision will make a great game out of getting thin!

I WILL MAKE IT FUN

To everything there is a season,
A time for every purpose under heaven:
A time to weep, And a time to laugh; A time to mourn,
And a time to dance.
(ECCLESIASTES 3:1, 4 NKJV)

I never thought I could weave fun and laughter into the dreariness of diet. Everybody knows that diets are a time of seriousness and anxiety—a big drag. You're supposed to suspend fun and willingly be miserable, just like every other good dieter. Diets are a time of weeping and mourning over food you won't get to eat, your scale which refuses to budge, and the menacing temptation which surrounds you. You're expected to have pursed lips—not to be *laughing your head off.*

Make it fun? It never occurred to be that *anything* about weight loss might be fun.

The *right time to diet* was only if I had a vacant calendar with no scheduled social activity—*no scheduled fun.* All fun was supposed to be officially cancelled *until the weight was lost.*

But for me, *the weight was never fully lost.* Social occasions and events always interrupted my plan. Maybe it's just *my* family and friends, but our good times always include food. Whenever it is *a time to laugh* and *a time to dance*, it's also *a time to eat.*

I'd bravely start a diet on a Monday *(of course)*, planning to reject any opportunity for fun and give my *undivided attention* to the wretched task of diet. All would go well for a day or two, until I'd get a call from a friend, and … well, *you* know the story. It's your story, too.

Weight loss takes time—*much more time than I had* between weddings, family events, banquets, holidays, birthdays, business trips, ministry events, and dinners with friends. My husband and I share a huge family. I have more close friendships than anyone deserves. I love too many people; I care about too many causes to have enough time left over for something as dreary, draining and *un-fun* as *weight loss.*

If only I could be left alone, I thought. *So I could diet.*

I decided I'd either have to *enter a monastery—or else figure out a way to make it fun.*

Then it hit me. *Wait a minute! The time to mourn is over! Back when overeating held me in its merciless grip and I was enslaved to appetite… that was the time to weep and mourn. But now? On my joyride to thin? Now is a time to laugh… a time to dance.*

I made the wise decision to make it fun, to turn the daily grind of diet into a sporting event. I resolved to bring laughter into the process of losing weight, to infuse a spirit of fun and celebration into every single day. *And* to incorporate my *social calendar* into *a game* that takes me to thin. *It worked!*

I made up a game, and then another. Over time, I learned

to make little games out of ordinary accountability, out of reminders, out of getting on the scale and setting goals and evaluating obstacles. *I turned weight-loss into a pastime, its process into playtime.* No longer did I just weigh a food. Now I called out "pop quiz!" and guessed the ounces first. No longer were my cryptic internet passwords boring. Now were all hilarious reminders of my current goal. No longer did my calendar pop-up only with appointments. Now I also scheduled a daily prompt of playful motivation.

After I made the decision to make it fun, my life became more fun. And more thin.

Approached lightheartedly, my little games breathed new life and *happy passion* into my weight-loss plan. *Passion increases with play,* so I playfully engaged my inner child. Even my accountability structures became pleasurable. *Fun really is a state of mind.*

Then, something crazy-good happened. After I made the decision to *make it fun,* my *life* became more fun. *And more thin!*

GAMES

We enjoy games. They entertain us. The right games also *grow* us.

Games create energy toward a specific outcome. You can start a game with your mind scattered on a million things, but within moments, there is only *one* thing: *your next move.*

Games create happiness. When you're in the midst of an absorbing game, an endorphin-like high envelops you. Games add glee and focused energy with every single move. Fun shows on the face. It looks like youth! I've never seen a person play a game and look sad at the same time.

Games create immediate energy, buzz, and heightened awareness. They fill us with a sense of power as we sharpen our strategy and outsmart our obstacle. Games give us a thrill as we push past our challenges to win our victory.

Have you ever noticed that when you really get into playing a game, another persona takes over? We all have a *game-warrior personality*. A good game sends us into a nearly hypnotic state of *happy focused striving*. Energy and passion arise from we-don't-know-where.

When you make weight loss a game, the very *process* of weight loss becomes fun and absorbing; a *thinking* game, like chess, in which you *delight* in outsmarting your opponent...except the opponent is *also you!* It's exciting *and* relaxing, all at the same time.

The Game of Games

I believe that throwing down a *special challenge* is the game of all games. The impact of *this one game* on your energy, momentum and staying power is nothing short of astonishing.

A short-term special challenge generates fresh excitement and specific direction for *right-now-this-minute*. It infuses you with brand new sporting energy. Best of all, it causes *an amazing reversal of diet procrastination*.

A special challenge automatically reshapes your *response* to stress. It trades your former *stress* response for a *game response*, replacing former frustration with fun. The power is in its process—a process leading directly to *thin*.

During one of my special challenges, I had a *really* bad day and was in a state of deep distress. Sniffling through tears and pre-wired to eat, *yet I did not eat*. I didn't even *think* about eating. Why? *I was in the middle of my "Hot Wife Challenge," and I wanted to win the game!*

Never have I seen anything work as well as a special challenge. *Not ever!*

After I made the decision to make it fun, I *forgot* I was on a diet. *I thought I was just trying to win a game!* I'm just a warrior princess! Yes, it's all in your head. I'm thankful I've learned how to outsmart mine.

࿔

Throwing down a special challenge will keep you from postponing or interrupting weight loss due to your impossible calendar. *People will no longer be a problem.* In fact, it will become a game to overcome social obstacles of thin.

Let's peek into a scene from one of my many successful special challenges. Then I'll explain the interesting components of this most valuable game.

THE CHIP-FEST

It was a happy weekend. A wonderful crowd of beloved company surrounded the kitchen counter, on which they descended like pelicans on a bountiful basket. The prize catch? An array of chips, dips and goodies including two kinds of potato chips, tortilla chips, plus every flavor of Doritos ever made. What a generous host!

And the dips? Salsa, guacamole, spinach-artichoke and onion. There were also those yummy peanut butter-stuffed pretzels. It's a marvel that so much salt and fat can fit into one afternoon snack.

I was that host. *And I skipped the chip-fest.* I stayed ten feet away, and from that safe distance I contentedly smiled and chatted as my visiting pelicans feasted.

Only one thing gave me the proud passion needed to bypass the chip-fest: I was in the middle of a game, fully absorbed with the happy prospect of winning it. I had thrown down a special challenge, was just four days from completion, and *I wanted to win the game* more than I wanted to eat chips and dip.

I can have a chip-fest any day I want. But I didn't want to have it *today*. The excitement and satisfaction of racing to win my game were too fabulous to spoil with ... chips.

Over the entire span of a diet, resisting the chip-fest would be difficult. But when you're only four days away from winning a special challenge, the thought of being bumped out of your game is far worse than skipping a few chips. *When a game mentality takes charge, it brings happy passion.* The thought of *anything coming between you and your win* becomes *unwanted* and unacceptable.

When you host company, you have to feed them differently than you feed just you. Depending on the company, very differently. But just four days from winning a special challenge, do chips tempt me? Are you kidding? If anything, the chips annoy me. Their presence at my table seems trivial and uninvited, like a mosquito. *I'm not interested.*

> *The naturally thin among us are so accustomed to the blessing of thin; they don't fully appreciate the intensity of joy and freedom that floods us when we attain it.*

On the day of the chip-fest, I did *not* forfeit gratification. Bound by diet? No, I was happily engaged in a *game*. I felt free, swapping a lesser thrill for a *lasting thrill*. I had a bigger yes inside me than the chip-fest. I made a bargain trade—ten minutes of *yum* for a thin life of *hum!* Yes, dear one. *Being thin feels that good. It feels even better than you dreamed it would.*

Old-style dieting is like striking a match that flickers when the chips hit the table, because a diet has no energy source of its own. But *fun* is a flame that keeps on burning, *even when you have company.* To eat a bunch of chips with just *four days left? Unthinkable!*

If I had joined the chip-fest, the world wouldn't end. I might have had an hour of temporary satisfaction, factoring in the fat grams hidden in the dips. But the satisfaction of *thin* stays with me every waking hour. Its endorphin-like feeling is always present; it never goes away. It infuses my bloodstream with something better than chips: it infuses me with constant delight.

The *naturally thin* among us are so accustomed to the blessing of *thin;* they don't fully appreciate the intensity of joy and freedom that *floods* us when we attain it. But *we who were not always thin have a more profound appreciation* of the ever-present delight of *life lived in a thin body.* For us, it was not always that way.

I want to win, I thought as I considered my options that day. *I'm a winner. I keep winning. I'm so close.* I'd much rather *win a game* than eat a bunch of chips and dip that I can eat next week—or any other time I want *except today.*

An empowering postscript: An hour later, everybody was hungry again! They were picking around, looking in the refrigerator, and thinking about food, while I, the *unchipped,* felt stable and serene, looking forward to our upcoming dinner.

Afterward, we all went out for a great restaurant meal. Know what? I think I enjoyed mine most. Feel the blessed truth and freedom of that. You can have that freedom, too.

Make a wise decision to make it fun, and you'll find playful passion to effortlessly get through the chip-fests in your life.

THE MAGIC FORMULA
FOR A SUCCESSFUL SPECIAL CHALLENGE

Let's explore the interesting mechanics of this amazing game, so you can play it to win.

Throw down a special challenge

First, throw down a red-hot-relevant challenge for a very short, intense period of time. Then do this...

Name your special challenge

Add a burst of fun. Give your challenge a great name. Make it funny and relevant: it should make you laugh out loud. The more ridiculous, personal, and outrageous a name, the better. For *maximum motivation,* it should be so silly, you'd hardly admit it to anyone. Around our 21st wedding anniversary, I threw down a special challenge. Did I name it *The Anniversary Challenge?* No...I went for zany, silly, laughable. I named it *The Hot Wife Challenge.* Do you see? The name should make you laugh!

Set a low goal

Wait. Did I say *low? Oh yes.* Why, your goal should be so low, you'd be downright embarrassed if you didn't win. So low, *the worst dieter in the universe* could *easily achieve it!*

I know—this is not what you've heard before. But this is *very smart game strategy* that almost guarantees you the energizing fun of a win. Remember, a goal has no power to make weight loss happen faster. *A big goal doesn't indicate you want it more.* But any goal you set that you don't also *achieve* has disconcerting power to discourage and to destroy your confidence. *You can't let that happen!*

So give yourself a really good chance to win the game, and virtually no chance to fail. Winning is fun and will keep you motivated. *It's just plain smarter to set up a series of little wins than of big impossible goals you are forced to abandon.*

Early on, I threw down a 24-day challenge, with the goal of losing just *one pound* in about three and one-half weeks. How's *that* for a low goal?

I started the challenge on the day my husband was scheduled for knee replacement surgery. There would be three days at the hospital, followed by three weeks of post-op care at home. Just six weeks earlier, I had made my first of the 10 Wise Decisions. For the next 24 days, my brand new food and fitness routines were about to be tossed out the hospital window.

I won my 24-day challenge. I had highly focused direction and crystal clear purpose for those chaotic 24 days. The challenge gave me an energizing path to follow—*instead of an excuse to drop out of my weight-loss plan.* Winning the challenge gave me joy. It greatly increased my confidence and *assured* me I really could live a thin lifestyle.

For special challenges, I define all *wins* as *completing the game within one pound of goal.* I have an affectionate term for it: I call it a *grace pound. My grace pound has helped me win many challenges!*

For this particular challenge, my master scorecard says I *completed within one pound of goal.* I think you know what that means! I didn't lose a single pound in those 24 days. Maybe I really am the worst dieter in the universe. *But I won the game!*

Let's unpack this carefully. I checked off this challenge *as a successful completion,* although I did not lose even the single hoped-for little pound. But I did maintain my weight, despite a very difficult 24 days—during which our beloved dog, whose health had been failing, passed away.

You set the rules. Set them in a way that makes you a winner!

I know what you're thinking: *Why throw down a special challenge at a time like that?* But what if I hadn't? There is no telling how much weight I would have *gained* during that tough period.

What would have happened if I had set my goal too high? I would have quit. I would have abandoned my special challenge (and probably all weight loss) as *not a good idea at this time*. That would have added to my sorrows.

Because my goal was so low *(lose only one pound),* I stayed fully engaged. I never had to do much more than maintain some semblance of healthy, lighter eating. *That meant that on bad food days—of which I had plenty—I was never discouraged into giving up.* There was always hope to win the game. I had reason to stay the course.

> *Because my goal was so low, I stayed fully engaged.*

The game worked perfectly. My special challenge gave me extra energy to get through those difficult weeks. Strategizing and walking through my win was fun and empowering and readied me for the next one! See how the proper formula makes the difference? *Tiny goals = momentum, engagement, empowerment, confidence.*

I start each special challenge with a *tiny* goal and a *big* sassy attitude—and I *complete* it with giggly energy, *because I always win*. Winner, winner, winner, again and again. Energized by my little victories, my weight-loss became a constant game in which I got smaller and smaller.

I'm such a winner. *And so are you.*

Set your dates

Each special challenge should be unique and specific to your *calendar*. Choose a start and stop date that sticks out as being particularly relevant. Remember, *thin* does not start on a Monday. *Thin* isn't relegated to exact calendar weeks. Your special challenge might start on a Thursday and go 11 days until just before or after your big event. Set each special challenge around the truth of your personal schedule so it can provide energy and focus exactly when you need it most.

That December, I did a 22-day special challenge with the goal of losing two pounds *over Christmas*. I carefully noted my expected obstacles: holiday goodies, parties, and big, wonderful holiday meals. My calendar was crazy, and we all know it's *the worst month to diet*. But because I had thrown down a challenge, I had no discouragement or fear. I never went off course, so *I never had to re-start*. Though still experiencing deep grief over the loss of my dog, I felt a sense of confident purpose toward getting thin. *My energy for thin renewed itself daily.* I knew that each day was part of something more hopeful and significant than just getting through it. *Tiny* goals allowed me to be flexible and comfortable in my eating at those times when *I just needed more.* The challenge itself kept me pleasantly distracted with a very short term, attainable goal, which *was always within just a few days.* The short time to completion gave me an opportunity to feel accomplished and confident. Guess what? A week after my great-big-Christmas dinner, *I completed the challenge. I won the game.*

A month later, I was scheduled for three out-of-town trips, with flight and hotel stays—plus jury duty. Talk about a diet buster! So, I planned a 28-day special challenge around them. One trip was a five-day retreat for writers where they served only heavy southern cooking and incredible desserts. I was really concerned about this, as there would be *no other food options available.* Then still overweight, my goal was to lose one pound during the *entire* four-week challenge. *Thanks to my low goal, I completed my challenge. I won the game! A full week early.*

As soon as you hit your goal, *game's over!* Take a few days break. But not too many days! Then make up a new special challenge!

Early on, I set my special challenges for up to a month. Then I discovered that a shorter challenge is more fun. Choose your duration carefully, with a well-defined start and stop, because once it stops engaging you, it is no longer a game. For me, ten to twenty days is just about perfect.

Strategize your obstacles

Strategy is the most fun part of a game. Carefully identify any social event or obstacle that will occur during your special challenge. *How* will you overcome it? How will you win? With smart, game-like strategy, that's how.

The obstacles create your game. Let your creative games-manship figure out a winning strategy to crash happily through each obstacle. The bigger they are, the more thrilling is your win. This all sounds nutty, and it is. But it works like nothing else I've ever seen. A special challenge is a *game,* and being in the middle of a game is wholly absorbing and fun.

You don't need to minimize your upcoming obstacles or pretend they won't affect you. *No exaggerated commitments or broken promises for you!* Not anymore. Those only made you feel weaker. Identify your obstacles and strategize around them, always with gentleness toward yourself.

Some weight loss obstacles on your calendar are worthy, like a wedding or family event. Others are just annoying obligations, tests of your will and disruptions to your pleasing new food-style.

Don't worry. *Identifying* obstacles won't make you *negative*. It will make you *creative*. The obstacles *define* your strategy. Identify every potential hindrance, every threat to thin—*and then slam it with creative advance strategy*.

For the writer's retreat, I had a very specific strategy ready-to-go; *a strategic path to follow*. There's no way I could have won that special challenge otherwise. Once creatively strategized, my mission had clarity and was *fun*. I came home confident and proud of myself.

Keep a permanent scorecard

I keep a master scorecard, so when I begin a special challenge, *I know it is going to count.* Mine is written in ink, *with no option to erase*. I can't make it go away. Win or lose, the result is going to be a permanent part of my *personal stats*. I'm certain that my scorecard is a big part of why I always do so well on every single challenge.

My scorecard means so much to me for other reasons, too! It documents my success in navigating my life, not just my *weight*. I post *all* my special challenges for the *whole year* onto one master scorecard. For me, it becomes a kind of grown up *honor roll*, giving me the confidence and courage I need to take on even greater pursuits. My scorecard results assure me *I keep faith with self.* And that I can be trusted to *do* what I *promise*.

> *To increase your fun and maximize your weight loss, learn and practice the art of celebration.*

CELEBRATE!

When was the last time you celebrated anything about *you?* To increase fun *and* maximize weight loss, learn and practice the art of *celebration.*

To celebrate is to *observe, honor, praise, mark, or proclaim.* Celebration isn't necessarily an *activity,* it's an *attitude.* It's an intentional response of joy for the little blessings in your life. Celebration feels good. You've felt mine throughout these pages. *Celebrate everything:* the signing of your 10 Wise Decisions, your little processes, *and your every little win.* Celebrate your two minutes on the treadmill, or that you threw the last bite of the cookie away. *Celebrate constantly.*

Celebration is appreciation. It's an intentional pause to honor what God did in your life, what your creator allowed to happen for you.

Celebration is healthy. It digests life's blessings.

Celebration is humble. It looks up.

Celebration is thankfulness. It's your little thank-you gift to God.

Celebration is forward-looking and growth-oriented. It resets your achievement bar higher.

Celebration is biblical, part of Jesus' first public miracle. (SEE JOHN 2:1–11.)

Celebration is ordained. It is "a time to laugh" and "a time to dance."

Celebration exalts God.

✧

Some people aren't very skilled at celebration. How tired they must be. They stay in striving mode and never take—or give to others—a well-deserved *pause* to *celebrate*. Has it been that way for you? No wonder you get tired of trying!

Lack of celebration decreases energy. When you withhold closure for small accomplishments, energy wanes and weariness increases. So, pause and celebrate every little victory along your joyful ride to thin, for without *close-out* of your accomplishments, you'll *burn-out*. Caution: *For the un-thin, burn-out is dangerous.*

And there's something else. When we don't acknowledge and celebrate our victories, it's *as if* we're ungrateful to God.

Dear one, please don't wait any longer. Celebrate *now*... and one day you'll celebrate *thin!*

PRAYER JOURNAL ENTRY

I can't believe it. I'm just thrilled. This is what I dreamed to reach by next month, not before! I even love all the wonderfully silly complications of thin, such as having to get rid of clothes because they are just too big. Oh my. Thank you, Father. Now let me help others.

I love to occupy myself with the *playful pleasures of thin*. Fun games of *thin* fill my life, my mind, and my calendar. *Fun has made the ride to thin enjoyable.* I've noticed that since I'm on a fun ride, *I no longer ask when I can get off.*

Starting today, do everything you can to make it fun. Make a *game* out of weight loss, and *you will lose your weight.*

Best of all, when you arrive at your goal—and I know you will—you'll already know exactly how to stay there—relaxed, happy, and highly experienced at meshing your social calendar with your thin lifestyle.

So move over, Candy Crush Saga. *A new game's in town!* It's time to create your very own *Fat Crush Saga.*

Let the games begin...

✧

My 7ᵀᴴ Wise Decision
I Will Make it Fun.

Signature _____ Date _____

Next: Our 8ᵗʰ Wise Decision breaks the back of the stronghold of food!

I WILL FAST

Empty yourself. Then refill...

A *hh, fasting.* A wonderful concept *for other people,* for those whose stomachs don't hurt all the time, like mine did. Never did I imagine I would have the ability to fast, not for a single meal. I had the perfect excuse: a history of ulcers dating back to age 14. Case closed. Or so I thought.

But I also had a dilemma.

I knew that if I were ever going to break the stronghold of food that had plagued me and generations of family before me, I would need to be infused with superpower. The Bible says that to break this kind of stronghold requires prayer and fasting (SEE MATTHEW 17:21). When it feels as if super glue has attached a particular sin to your life, a sin like overeating that is so deeply embedded and seemingly unbreakable, there is but no other way to freedom than by fasting.

Some strongholds begin as an innocuous, just-this-once sin. We eat too much, *just this once.* It feels good. And becomes a habit. The habit becomes a lifestyle, which becomes a life, and eventually a generational destiny. The stronghold may have started in childhood. Or even before. It might have formed *generations ago* and been passed down to us. Until it is broken, and I mean *shattered*, it will become part of our own legacy to beloved generations that follow.

I did not fast to win God's love or favor. I knew I already had both.

Willpower alone cannot break an overeating stronghold. A mere diet applied against it is puny and will eventually fail. Although *diet* applies great pressure, it applies it to the wrong place. If you apply a tight compression bandage to your *leg* to stop profuse bleeding originating in your *arm*, then no amount of force, pressure or effort by you will stop your arm from bleeding.

There is nothing wrong with diets, and Lord knows we sometimes need them. But they are seldom enough, for they focus on the *symptoms* of overweight and not the *cause*.

To apply a diet to a *stronghold* is to apply mighty pressure *to the wrong thing.* What we really need is to break the spiritual stronghold that has kept us locked in a magnetic force-field with food. *Through fasting, we can break that stronghold.*

A spiritual fast is a *spiritual* act for a *spiritual* purpose. It is *not* a diet—and *not* a punishment or penance for overeating. Its purpose is to open yourself to a mighty unleashing of spiritual strength and power in your life.

I did not fast to win God's love or favor. I knew I already had both. After making my wise decision to live life loved, I was even more aware of his love for me. Now I wanted to give him more of my heart, with no portion of my affection held in reserve for my *other* secret love: food. I wanted to wrench myself free to pursue my highest dreams, with no portion of my life held in bondage to *anything*.

So I resigned my fear of fasting and made my next wise decision. *I will fast a meal. The stronghold will stop here. That's it. It will end with me.*

PRAYER JOURNAL ENTRY:

I don't want to be ruled by appetite, Lord. Unless it's an appetite for you in my life.

༚

Several thin friends urgently warned me against fasting. They were concerned it would slow my weight loss. *That may or may not be true,* I responded patiently. *But God is more important to me than my weight. And I'm doing this for him.*

What my well-meaning friends didn't realize was that without fasting—without dislodging the *root of my weight problem*—there could be no permanent weight loss for me. I would forever be *hooked* on food. Even if I dieted my heart out, I would ultimately remain un-thin.

My decision to fast had nothing to do with *food!* It was a *spiritual* decision to enter a fierce battle against an unseen stronghold of overeating, a battle *I intended to win*. This would be a war of an *invisible* kind, so I would need *invisible* weapons *not* of this world. Until I rid my house (my body) of strongholds, oppressive cravings, and an ungodly attraction to food, I would never be free of weight issues.

I had already made my wise decision to finish having a weight problem. In order to finish, I would have to fast. It was as simple as that.

The World's Wisdom

The world's evolutionist "wisdom" is for us to go around eating every two or three hours, as we supposedly did when we were animals foraging in the jungle. They say we should eat about six times a day. Six *tiny little meals.*

Are they kidding? To instruct someone with a weight problem to go to the refrigerator six times a day for a *tiny little meal* is like instructing someone with a drinking problem to go to a local bar six times a day and *order only water.*

Yet we, the overweight, are expected to choose only a celery stick and two slices of apple. Or a small protein bar. You know exactly what will happen: The small health bar will go missing and be replaced by a big chocolate bar. The celery stick will be eaten, followed by a donut—like everybody else at the office is eating.

This all-day grazing concept may be harmless to a naturally thin person who has no magnetic attraction to food or to an athlete in training. But to an overeater? We are trying to make food *less* of a focus, *not more.*

Realistically, how often can we go to our food equivalent of a local bar and *order only water?*

When I carefully contemplated the popular trend of eating every few hours, I found a number of ways in which it conflicted with my personal dream of thin.

I do not want to be someone who constantly needs to eat. Life is about more than food.

I do not want to eat while doing other activities. Riding in the car should not include eating.

When working, I do not want to have to stop repeatedly for food. I don't even want to think about food. And I want to feel proud about that!

When traveling, I do not want to have to make special accommodation for my continually needy stomach, as I've had to do on every vacation of my life.

When at an all-day event, I do not want to be the one who has to sneak out of the room between lunch and dinner for my snack.

When I am a houseguest and food is not under my control, I do not want to have to carry it in my luggage or be unnecessarily focused on the longings of my stomach.

Six meals a day *necessitates mindless eating!* How counterproductive is that? Few among us have the time and space to turn off the whole world while we prepare, *chew mindfully,* and clean up six personal meals per day. I don't. Do you?

In general, I do not want to be the person known for chewing all the time. I am not a cow; I am a productive woman. I want to *do,* not to *eat.* I want to *be,* not to *eat.* I want to *live,* not to *eat.*

So this fad of constant eating is definitely *not* for me. *Oh, you protest, it's only a protein bar!* Well, I hate to be the one to tell you, but a protein bar is not *real food.* It did not grow in the ground. It never swam in the water. It never roamed on the range. It was made in a factory and comes to you in a plastic wrapper. How much fabricated false-food do you really want to put into your body?

LOVE RELATIONSHIPS

By fasting, I also sought to reorder the priority of my love relationships. I began to reflect on who and what would receive *the gift of my love.* I had been excessively ardent toward food, which did not love me. And complacent toward God who did. I would stop loving food, which has no ability to love me back. I wanted more of God and (quite literally) less of me.

God had been high on my *who-have-I-been-taking-for-granted* list. No more. I would be more circumspect regarding who and what would receive the gift of my ardent devotion.

☙

For years, thin friends had been giving me books on fasting. I did read them, though I never planned to actually fast. Some were really good; their sincerity and wisdom touched me. After reading, I patted them affectionately, like a little dog I don't want on my lap. I like you. Now go away. Not now.

Then one day I cleaned out my bookcase. There it was, *The Diet Alternative* by Diane Hamilton (Whitaker House, 1984). The pages were yellowing. I looked at the cover. *When did I get this? Why hadn't I seen this before?*

I've always said that you can *read a book and change your whole world.* Of all the great books I had read on fasting, this one touched me the most. I have no recollection of actually buying or receiving the book. How providential that I found this buried little treasure of words at just the right time. It was a tiny jewel of a message in a simple paperback wrapper, its pages weathered by nearly 30 years and over a dozen house moves. What a miracle it survived the give-away box. How thankful I am that it did.

Diane Hamilton's book empowered me because she spoke of fasting *just one meal per day:* lunch. She noted that in the Bible, when God fed the Israelites in the desert, he provided a morning and evening meal, but there was no biblical mention of lunch.

Hmmm, I wondered. My sensitive, acid stomach usually growled by 11 am. Could I make it to five? And do I want to?

But I *did* want to. I wanted to do it for the Lord. And for my weight. I wanted to push past *me*.

I reviewed some guidelines for a *spiritual* fast. Fasting is not merely the absence of eating. It is of spiritual benefit only if it is spiritually approached. If your business meeting runs late and forces you to skip lunch, that doesn't qualify as a spiritual fast. If you aren't hungry today (unlikely as that is), and didn't eat, neither is that a spiritual fast. If your doctor tells you not to eat before a medical procedure, neither is that a spiritual fast.

In a spiritual fast, you sincerely seek to exalt God above your unrelenting appetite for a very brief and finite period of time. Wow.

A spiritual fast is intentional, specific, set in advance and dedicated to God. You commit *in advance* to potential discomfort of body in order to seek spiritual gain. Therein lies its power: the surrendered will of a self-gratifying mortal. In a spiritual fast, you sincerely seek to exalt God above your unrelenting appetite for a very brief and finite period of time. Wow.

Diane's book melted away the last of my fear and resistance. *All right,* I exhaled. *I will try this impossible business of fasting. I will fast lunch.*

And so I began.

꽃

All set for my big day, I was a little nervous and more than a little excited. Hopeful that I could endure it, I was ready for God to replace my worn-out will. Bracing against a hunger that I feared might be intolerable, I made the decision to let go— just this one day—for the nine hours between breakfast and dinner. I would surrender that precious meal that mattered so much to me: my lunch.

Following a super-large, high-protein breakfast and well-armed for the day with apple juice, emergency crackers, and plenty of water, I dedicated in advance to God all the hunger I expected between breakfast and dinner. Then I waited.

Funny how mixed up I was back then. I used to *fear* what is good (short-term hunger) and *celebrate* what is not good (being stuffed). I was about to discover *the exquisite joy of less*. If you want beauty, power, holiness, deliverance, and health, look no further. Nothing beats a one-meal fast.

Clean hunger—holy hunger—is in a joy-class so sacred,
it feels like it should be available by prescription only.

Clean hunger is one of the most delightful feelings you will ever experience. No kidding! The likely reason you have feared hunger is because you've had "scary hunger," that low-blood-sugar angst associated with shakiness, dizziness, headaches, and nausea. We've confused real hunger with low blood sugar for so long; we don't remember what real hunger feels like. Low blood sugar is the *fake imitator* of true hunger; it hits you after high-sugar intake. The ultimate ricochet, no one would willingly endure that. I don't think it would even be safe to try!

I was about to discover the exquisite joy of less.

Clean hunger, on the other hand, is actually *pleasant*. It's peaceful, not fearsome. It's physically healthful and empowering, emotionally strengthening and spiritually cleansing. There is something about an empty stomach that invites alertness, awareness, and attention.

Fasting lunch on most weekdays is what broke the back of my stronghold. It also readied me for a wonderful blessing I didn't know would be delivered to my door about six weeks later.

PRAYER JOURNAL ENTRY

You answered my prayer when I called out to you in sorrow and grief over my weight. You gave me fresh inspiration.

You strengthened me to try fasting, to break the stronghold of food and eating in my life.

You made my stomach okay.

You gave me the will to do your good pleasure.

You took me smoothly and quickly from overweight to normalcy, just two days before my sister's gift of clothing would arrive.

You gave me the dignity and GOD-fident honor of having them all fit. Every one of them fit. No shame. No loss of esteem. They all fit.

THE EXQUISITE BLESSING OF HUNGER

At a certain point in the afternoon of a lunch fast, you will realize your stomach is empty. Not ill, not even hungry, just empty. Invite that feeling of emptiness, appreciate it, and embrace it. No matter your temporary present weight, you'll feel a fresh breeze of leanness—a rightness that floods your being. To me, an empty stomach now feels sacred. An overfed stomach feels awful.

I always eat a high-protein snack mid-morning, right after the gym. So some of my fasts are shorter than others. On mornings I have breakfast by 7 am, I begin to be aware of emptiness by 2 pm. It's a self-empowering sensation, a confidence generator.

About an hour *after emptiness* comes the exquisite awareness of *actual hunger.* I smile at the first signal of clean hunger, knowing I am entering a sacred place.

3:32 pm. It's starting. That feeling—it wells up inside, and I nod affirmatively at no one, for I am alone in the house. It feels good. *Hello, Lord.*

This is an ideal time for a quick prayer break. When I feel holy hunger, the kind I've *earned via a deliberate decision to empty myself before God,* I enter into an incredible place of sweet spiritual intimacy, unlike anything I've ever known. I can compare it to nothing else.

4:01 pm. My stomach is empty. I feel…confident. My identity and esteem swell with newfound power, rightness, and health. It feels so good. I like who I am becoming. At last I am becoming the woman I long to be.

I begin to feel the flow of a loving connection from within me toward those nameless men and women around the world who experience hunger every day. And to their children. Oh, to their children. How could I have mindlessly overeaten while their growing bodies have gone without food? God loves them—and he loves me, too. They do not have enough, and I have too much.

Now I am joyfully *one with them* for at least these few sacred hours. I am eating *within my means,* aware of God's other beloveds, and not just me. My focus thoughtfully expands; those brief hours of hunger are a perfect time to become other-centered.

Joyful hunger lasts just a short time, perhaps two or three hours. Then, at some point, the gnawing calls out a bit more intently, and my focus returns to me. Unlike my brothers and sisters around the world, I do not have to withstand hunger beyond a certain rather puny point, usually just until 6 o'clock. Then, with a blend of sadness and relief, I let go of those sacred, set-apart hours and again fill myself with food. With my fast now over, I celebrate another victory of personal growth and freedom. On those days I fast lunch, dinner tastes especially satisfying.

I consider my lunch fast *fulfilled* at 5 pm, though dinner doesn't come until later. If needed, I have a light snack to break the fast. When you fast, you write the rules, but you must write them in advance.

God knows my heart, so I fast *gently,* with several pre-written *allowables* to compensate for my less-than-perfect bodily processes. These are what gave me the courage to try fasting the first time:

1. A container of apple juice, *if* I feel the least shaky or want it for any reason.

2. A small handful (about five) gluten-free crackers, intentionally of a type I do *not* especially like. They whisk away any hint of physical discomfort other than pure hunger. This is the only chewing I allow myself.

3. Chicken or vegetable broth, if needed.

I try to designate many weekdays to this most sacred *privilege* of fasting lunch. But I never plan a fasting day too far in advance or without carefully considering my schedule and my stomach. It is unwise to make a rash promise to God.

Breakfast, especially before a lunch fast, is high-protein and hearty, including a small amount of high-fiber grain. I usually choose half a high-fiber English muffin, toasted twice, heaped high with my protein of choice: peanut butter, tuna salad, or scrambled eggs. Crunchy and yummy. All this and a glass of fat-free milk, too. After the slow ingestion of 350—400 calories into a stomach already well-hydrated with water, I'm all set for six or seven hours of reasonable comfort.

> *If like me, you work and want accelerated mental acuity, try brief periods of fasting. It is so cleansing, so powerful; it's almost an altered state!*

With this kind of breakfast, you needn't fear fasting. If like me, you work and want accelerated mental acuity, try brief periods of fasting. It is so cleansing, so powerful; it's almost an altered state!

Support your fasting with many additional glasses of water. When fasting, stay very well hydrated.

At noontime, when others are eating lunch, I distract myself by doing *non-food* activities like shopping or running errands, or tackling special projects. I now have the gift of being able to focus more on *life,* and less on *food. Stronghold shattered!*

One oddity about fasting, and a reason I know God is in it, is that on days I fast, I receive supernatural ability to live and work alongside unfulfilled hunger. Contrast that to the days I *don't* commit to fast, when my lunchtime hunger is strong enough to make me wonder how I ever fasted at all.

♧

Fasting is something I never dreamed I could do. But I did. *And if your doctor says yes*, you can do it too. Fasting serves as an on-ramp to a highway leading most directly to the thin life you want. Fasting trades your miserable, old strongholds for wonderful new beginnings.

As you empty yourself of the worst of you, you break the back of your stronghold. God supercharges and refills that space with power, love, and a sound mind. It is overwhelming how spiritual fasts can change your life.

After fasting, I changed. Oh, how I changed. Fasting introduced me to one of the sweetest experiences one can ever know: *the intimate joy of prayerful hunger.* There is absolutely nothing like it.

I've had a distinct lessening of the inner pull toward certain foods, including those that formerly inspired ecstasy. Food has lost its power. Weight loss is no longer a process of gritted teeth or clenched hands, but *a miraculous release* of the possessive grip of the fork. Fasting ushers in a more gracious attitude toward food and eating that makes weight loss downright easy. Less really *is* more. I find the taste of food sweeter when there is a bit less of it in my otherwise well-fed day.

GLORY

You don't want to miss the glory of hunger. There is power within it like I've never before experienced. In that sweet, empty place before God, I can say wholeheartedly, *he is Lord of all.* In my hunger, I feel gratitude and humility, knowing that unlike starving innocents around the world, I do have a choice. I have chosen hunger, by my own will, for a very brief and finite amount of time.

Fasting is a demonstration that our love for the Father, and for ourselves, is greater than our love for food. And that we really do trust him to fill us again.

Dear one, live; don't eat. Don't let food continue to be the focus of all your days. *Make friends with the hunger you've feared.* Honest hunger won't hurt you; it will *free* you.

Make a courageous and life-changing decision to fast a meal. Try it once, and be awakened! Rejoice!

My 8ᵗʰ Wise Decision

I Will Talk With My Doctor, and If Medically Approved, I Will Fast a Meal.

Signature _____ Date _____

Next: Learn to utilize the hidden power of your "seventh sense"!

GOD-SENSE

A life of faith un-interrupted.

Sight, sound, smell, taste, and touch. I appreciate my senses. I just don't want to be *ruled* by them. Clearly, my five were on *sensory overload!* At mealtimes, they were so highly sharpened on food, that they were dulled to spirit. I set out to *reverse* that.

I generally start most days at a spiritual level. But I noticed that once I entered the *outside* world, my *inside* spirit seemed to *close for business* for the rest of the day. Once my five senses were engaged, they took over completely.

I lacked God-sense.

My senses were alarmingly overstimulated by the very nearness of food. They needed to somehow be demagnetized. My mealtime mission was to begin to heighten my sensation of *God* over *food.* If I was ever going to honor God with my *body,* I would have to stay connected to his "radio frequency," *even during lasagna.* I wanted to learn to be dispassionate and detached from the fierce attractant of food, *even while I was eating it.*

The five temporal senses can be enjoyed with pleasant appreciation, with humor, and even with curiosity. But they are flawed. We are grateful to have them, but if we want to live a good life, a thin life, *we must master them.* Our five senses exist to serve us, and not we them. They are subject to us. We are their ruler. We must *never* bow down before them; *never* grant to our untrustworthy senses control of our destiny! Sovereignty over our senses is one decision the evil one doesn't want us to make.

My senses were alarmingly overstimulated by the very nearness of food.

I came up with a 5-part action plan to increase my God-sense by subduing the other five.

SIGHT

I decided to avoid looking at food unnecessarily. I would consciously dull my attraction to glossy photos in recipes, on television commercials, and in magazines. I would turn my eyes away from that which would destroy me. I would instead focus my gaze on the invisible and *fix my eyes* on what is unseen. I would be mature and attentive to the spiritual warfare occurring all around us.

SOUND

I would learn what to tune in. And what to tune out. I would stop listening to sabotaging self-talk rooted in futile worldly systems, or in harmful repetition of my low expectations. *I would not let the sound of food be a trigger for my soul.* I am not a dog who responds to a can opener; I am a child of God. I would listen for him, for the amazing way of escape he whispers in moments of indecision or temptation. From now on, I would listen for the sound of God within my spirit. I would let him tell me when to eat, *and when to stop eating.* Just as a mother can easily discern the cry of her own child in a room full of crying babies, so would I learn to *discern God's impression* over all the food-stimuli competing for my attention. Classic God-sense!

SMELL

I resolved to dull my sense of smell. I decried its former power over me, and I willed myself to become *unresponsive to its calling.* My olfactory gland would no longer control any element of my life. I would learn to live gently and harmoniously with food aroma, allowing sweet food fragrance to exist alongside me without having dominion over me. I would learn to appreciate the lovely smell of a bakery, without surrendering to it, and to be more sensitive to the sweet, wholesome fragrance of Christ within my life.

TASTE

I intended to dull my sense of taste, and even to *soften the glowing words* I formerly used to describe the taste of food on my tongue. From now on, I would permit food to *please me,* but not to *thrill me.* I would stop over-seasoning food and would begin to eat simply and lightly, with less excitement and less dependence on strong taste. Instead, I would taste and see that the Lord is good!

TOUCH

I would stop handling food so much, not "touch" food or fork so often, not walk around eating, and not allow my tongue to depend so constantly on the habit of touch. I would orally disengage, except at appropriate infrequent intervals. Instead, I would seek other kinds of touch. I would touch grace. Touch mercy. Touch the hem of his garment. Touch his glory.

☙

As I developed God-sense, I felt a remarkable lessening of the insistent tugs from the other five. My mealtime awareness of God grew more prominent as the urgency of the others seemed to fade. *Aware* of them, I was no longer *compelled* by them.

☙

One thing I've learned about my senses is that I don't have to allow them unrestricted influence over my eating. Now, I politely receive their capricious counsel (*That food smells wonderful!*) and their impetuous enthusiasm (*That cake looks gorgeous!*), but in a calm and dispassionate way. I practice being unresponsive to their chorus of unrestrained longing.

Once the five senses are demagnetized, you live in freedom. *This is how your thin friends live.* I now appreciate beautiful sights and smells, delectable sounds and tastes, and even the touch of food, with calmness and restraint.

PRIDE

Pride shuts down God-sense. And I had plenty of it. Because I was within twenty pounds of being normal weight and was essentially disciplined, my pride felt justified to me. *But it never is.* Masked as self-esteem, my pride did a lot to *make me feel good...* but did nothing to *make me thin.* Full of food, and proud for not being heavier than I was, I left no space for the humility I would need to figure out what exactly was stopping me from getting thin. Pride says, *I only overeat by a small amount.* But you know, dear one, it's still called a *bank robbery* even if you only take ten dollars.

SELF-SUFFICIENCY

Self-sufficiency was my ineffective substitute for God-sense. Every time I grow confident about my own sufficiency in matters of diet, I disappoint myself with a sudden new urge and desire for food. The self-appointed false god within me is utterly incapable of getting me to *thin.* I need the true God to escort me there.

Weight is an area of special weakness for me. Since I am his beloved child, my weakness is beloved to him. I now regard my own—and others'—weight weakness tenderly and without condemnation. God provides protection for me by inspiring boundaries, borders, and guardrails, along with some loving parental supervision. I, his beloved, cannot do this in my own strength. I cannot be the god of my own body. *I cannot get it right.*

For me, in this matter, I will always need God at front and center. Oh, I can imitate others who seem to be in easy control of their perfect weight. I can cast a jealous eye on their seeming spiritual independence in this matter of diet. They appear to have it all together. Thin comes so easily for them. But I know they have other issues, as does every man and woman on earth. The naturally thin among us are not superior; they need God's special touch in *other* areas that may be less visible than weight, areas in which they, too, are weak or damaged. But *my* issue is weight. That's where *I* need his touch—an extra layer of care and supervision, along with a big dose of guidance and forgiveness.

And I receive exactly what I need, provided generously,

without charge or judgment by my indefatigable God. He never tires of me; is never resistant to my need and has every resource instantly available when I call out to him. Talk about a diet guru! God-sense makes it almost laugh-out-loud easy. And the results? Miraculous.

Next: Our 9ᵗʰ Wise Decision will make thin last forever!

I WILL FINESSE

I will make thin last forever!

To *finesse* is to adapt when life goes off-script. This beautiful word describes a way of artfully managing your thin life. It hints of lightness of manner and elegant style. Finesse is all about diplomacy, delicacy, tact, and discreetness—knowing how to *gracefully* avoid embarrassment or distress.

When you live wholeheartedly in the 10 Wise Decisions, your *life* becomes gracefully elegant. The jagged edges and abrupt pivots between impulse and regret seem a distant memory. You no longer think in terms of fear, dread or consequences. Your food thoughts are increasingly peaceful—empowerment-based, not punishment-based—completely free of conflict. This is what freedom looks like—and how it lives.

You're slamming shut the door on shame and are reshaping the brand called *you*.

Make the wise decision to finesse. *Create a lifestyle of leanness that adapts to every situation.*

☙

A weight-loss plan starts out in a protected bubble, a temporary cocoon in which you shut out your ordinary routines and focus only on special foods and new ways of eating. At first, everything is just fine. Then the real world shows up, interrupting your tenuous new plan.

Reality soon bursts your bubble. An unexpected circumstance arises. You're needed here, you're needed there. Someone hurts your feelings. You're tired. A loved one has surgery. Focus distracted, attention diverted, at some point you take a much-needed time-out—and your wonderful weight-loss plan falls completely apart.

Confidence is shaken. *What happened?* You ask. *How can I fix it?* But there is no recovery strategy in place. So what do you do? You know exactly what you do. You give up. That's what I used to do, too.

But not anymore. *I made a wise decision that when life goes off-script, I will not falter. I will finesse.*

Sooner or later, life will rudely intrude on your plan to be THIN & BLESSED. If you don't finesse those unwelcome intrusions, you won't be able to get or stay thin.

But you needn't become a weight-loss casualty. You can make thin last forever, by practicing the interesting subtleties of your new, thin lifestyle. *You really can finesse.*

THE HABIT OF THIN

I live in a Florida neighborhood locally known as "horse country." Though I do not ride, I admire the elegant stateliness of horses as they stride down the streets near our home. The power of these magnificent animals is not displayed by their strength, speed, or size. No, their fame is due to the *elegance of their stride;* that exquisite coordination of muscle and intention as it thrusts forward gracefully. Now, that is beautiful! And powerful! When all the elements of their body coordinate in perfect harmony to move forward on a path, there is a *momentum* that is elegant, stately, even awe inspiring.

If a horse stumbles, it loses its momentum. Once momentum is stopped, it will takes a bit of time and conscious effort to recover its gliding cadence. Time subtracted. Effort added.

Habits are what set in motion a *graceful glide to thin, a momentum that keeps you in forward motion on the path to thin.* Momentum makes the thin life feel easy and natural.

Momentum makes the thin life feel easy and natural.

Your habits are the strong, silent type. Habits have the strength to make or break your thin future, but they do so in *silence*. Are your habits leading you toward—or away from—thin? Consider them carefully, for they *will not* call out their next move. *Observe* them—and *direct* them. Habits need supervision. *Leverage them to get exactly what you want.*

Is it your *habit* to open your refrigerator for no reason at all? To snack as you cook? To quickly clean your plate?

Or is it your *habit* to ignore the first impulse of hunger? To drink a glass of water before each meal? To watch the movie *without* food in hand?

Your best habits cause your best dreams to be actualized effortlessly. That's what momentum is all about. Habits exude a unique style of energy that is natural, straightforward, and evenly paced. The habit of thin is more valuable to you than money in terms of buying the outcome you want: *a thin body.*

Integrate habits of thin into your lifestyle and you'll find it almost impossible to fail. You will move methodically forward in the direction of your dreams with the same clip-clop rhythm as magnificent horses gliding on path. Clip-clop, clip-clop, each day moves you toward your lasting dream.

The momentum of those steps multiplies day by day,
until the rhythm of your habits becomes
the outcome of thin in your life.

Design your habits thoughtfully, embrace them affectionately. Delight in their sweet cadence as they glide you elegantly to thin. *Surrender them not* for vacation, company, or illness— not for *anything*. Cherish your best habits, and thank them for the magnificent and effortless power they provide you.

SACRED HABITS

Sacred habits are *cherished activities* regarded by you with reverence, dedicated to God, and immune from interference. A sacred habit is something you care *deeply* about doing. By restoring your balance, sacred habits help remove debris from your path to thin.

Do you have sacred habits, such as spending a few moments daily in prayer? Or do you pour yourself out to those around you, day after day, without regard to your own inner emptiness? When is the last time you inwardly *filled up* before outwardly *pouring out*? For how long has that inner warning light been flashing? And who will suffer most if you really do run out of gas?

B & B

My affectionate nickname for my most Sacred Habit is *B & B, my* code for "Bible & Breakfast." It's a daily special occasion. I eagerly arise early for it, set a place setting, sip tea, prepare a pleasing breakfast, dine rather than gulp, and have Bible and prayer time. All this before I exercise and begin my workday.

Time with God is my admission ticket to fresh discovery and sacred intimacy. It's how I connect the dots between need and want, between *true hunger* and *true fullness* in my life. I eat and drink heartily of God's Word, reminding myself that he is my portion and my cup. He is the Bread of Life. I who come to him will not hunger.

B & B brings harmony from the disparate components of my busy mind and busy life. Prayer time is an investment that unlocks my divine destiny, strengthens my will, and illuminates a timeless path I can trust and follow. During *B & B,* I examine and mend my ragged edges and redefine my borders, safe and secure. From *inner wholeness* comes *outer thinness.*

One of the B's stands for breakfast, which I usually attend to first, because I am hungry. Then, with emptied plate before me, *as a deliberate demonstration of leisure that I don't really have,* I open my prayer journal, pray, write a note to God about whatever inspires me, and read my Bible.

Some might think that combining eating with worship is irreverent or disrespectful. But I don't think it is disrespectful. *I think it is sweet.* What could be more natural or nurturing than having breakfast with one's Father?

Nurturing routines make the impossible, possible.

B & B establishes conversation and connection between Father and daughter at the start of the day. *It invites him to be a part of my eating experience,* not just a fast-mouthed prayer before the food gets cold. I love knowing that he is receiving the first-fruit of my earliest hours.

NURTURING ROUTINES

Live your beautiful life on purpose.

Nurturing routines do more than honor and safeguard weight loss. They also give you an almost unfair advantage to get and stay thin! They increase joy, elevate esteem, and boost confidence. It is astonishing how *thin* can be made possible for you via your nurturing routines. They are a great delivery system for the weight loss you crave; a wonderful launching point for *thin*.

My nurturing routines don't *bind* me. They *free* me, by allowing me to execute my *best*, rather than be ruled by my *worst*. *They make the impossible, possible.*

Routines are like white stripes on a wide highway. They keep me from wandering off course and wasting my thrilling opportunity to be thin.

Don't like routines? But your daily interaction with food is set to a dance of routine. We are cyclical beings, all of us; creatures of habit. We *like* to repeat ourselves. What satisfied you late last night, you will crave again tonight.

Off balance and toxic eating routines had been so woven into my lifestyle, I didn't even recognize them for what they were. But I've swapped those old criss-crossed patterns for wonderful new habits and nurturing routines.

☙

Routines allow you to escape argument with yourself. They plug the drain of self-sabotage and silence the whining voice of inner childish resistance.

Routines are masters of disguise. They dress up as willpower.

They give your highly focused resolve a much needed nap, as they propel you forward on precisely the right path, *even when you're not paying attention.* On those days your schedule and environment conspire against you, routines find a way. They are like the little-train-that-could, carrying you higher than you thought possible.

Your nurturing routines tell the world you are a person worth caring about, someone who values and self-stewards her life. As you demonstrate that you know how to care for your needs, you wordlessly settle any question that you can be trusted to care for the needs of others.

Routines never lie about love. *And the person they love is you.*

They are energy-savers. They save you the energy of decision-making.

They are tie-breakers. At times when one inner voice says yes, but another says no, they help you deliver on promises made to self.

They give your highly focused resolve a much needed nap, as they propel you forward on precisely the right path.

Routines are not rigid. They don't bind or constrict you to things you don't really want.

Routines are muscle-builders. They build the muscle of your intentionality.

They are escape artists that help you break out from old, ineffective patterns.

They keep safe that which you have prioritized. They protect that which you prize.

Routines are ballet bars for fluid, graceful expression of those values you hold dear. They are a means to a life elegantly lived, smooth and sure.

Successful routines are born from truth: *truth rearranged.* Design them cleverly, thoughtfully, *sensitively,* with respect for your lifestyle and regard for your preferences. They will give you immeasurable joy.

Please don't establish a routine to do what you have no intention of doing. Innocent routines were never intended to take the role of police enforcer. Create lovable routines you can absolutely hit out of the ballpark most of the time, *with just the smallest stretch.*

Successful routines must be personally authentic and true. You cannot adopt another person's routines. *If they are to empower you, they must fit you.* Just like a glove that is stretched but not forced.

⚘

Successful routines are flexible. Fixable. Disposable. If you have changed, outgrown them, or become bored, simply toss them away. As you practice, you'll enjoy new skill at creating your own nurturing routines. Meantime, if you accidentally create one that just isn't working for you, delete it. The worst thing you can do with a dysfunctional routine is drag it along and let it annoy you.

Remember: no more failure cycles for you anymore. Do what you must to protect your confidence. Change the game plan, tweak it, adjust it or rename it, *until the game itself helps you be a winner.*

Sleep

God wants his loved ones to get their proper rest. So sleep, my friend. Rest your full eight hours. The *un*-rested are often *un*-thin.

Protect your rest as best you can. You won't reach thin without it. Fatigue is a breeding ground for brokenness. I wonder how many broken weight-loss intentions are due only to fatigue.

Have you noticed the domino effect of insufficient sleep? First, you triage to figure out what scheduled tasks you might give up that day. Rushed and unrested, you mentally scan all you'd planned to do. First to go? *Exercise.* Next? *Spiritual time.* You can hardly think straight, no less pray and study. Productivity is compromised. Leisure, the truly valuable kind that renews and rejuvenates body and mind, is forsaken.

On especially tired days, how many extra calories would you guess you consume? I've heard 300 to 400 calories. And I believe it. More awake time means an additional meal or snack is likely, which will probably be carbohydrate-laden to meet your very real need for quick energy.

The *unrested* make *unfortunate* food choices. Your exhausted body seeks sugar to keep itself going. You are strangely attracted to carbs. At home, you lack fortitude to chop those vegetables for salad. In its place, you search through a fog of fatigue for that pizza-delivery menu.

Then there's that nasty little hormone called cortisol that triggers the mother of all enemies of thin: *your appetite.*

At a restaurant midweek, I saw a young, overweight woman in business attire having dinner with her children. *She's tired*, I thought. *I wish I could hug her.* I have a keen eye for tired-weight. I too lived tired for many years as I worked to build my business. As my success grew, unfortunately so did my dress size.

But there is something other than hard work that is also exhausting. *Overweight is an extremely tiring condition.* If you do nothing but get thin, you'll be surprised at how much more rested you feel—even with the same sleep habits and impossible schedule.

Examine your evening routines. Is whatever you do at night worth giving up a pant size? Maybe it is. Maybe you must. But maybe there's a creative way to slightly rework your schedule.

If you go to sleep at midnight, take baby steps to gently move toward a healthier sleep pattern. I used to go to sleep at around one a.m. Now my bedtime is ten pm sharp. It took a few *years* to get there, but I love my earlier bedtime. *And did I mention I got thin?*

Do not let anyone intimidate or discourage you by their low expectations based on their limited awareness.

Morning is joyful for the rested. When I arise early, the house is still. Even the sun is asleep. But God is not. I drink my favorite tea and pray for my favorite people. In the quiet, I listen for his prompting, his urging and his inspiration. I dream big dreams. And I write my heart out.

Please take extra care, dear one, to guard tonight. For everything you want for tomorrow will be impacted by tonight. *Your tomorrow is worth protecting!*

TACTLESS WORDS

To finesse means to sometimes tactfully dodge thoughtless or inappropriate words spoken to you. Be assured that the words of the tactless are not a curse on you! Do not receive them into your head or heart. If someone trivializes or ignores your obvious achievement or suggests your weight loss is temporary, *politely reject those words with a serene smile.* Do not let anyone intimidate or discourage you by *their* low expectations based on *their* limited awareness. Dear one, your plan is not their plan, your life is not their life, and your destiny is not their destiny.

Do you realize how extremely *difficult* it would be for you to gain back the weight? Why, you would have to *un-make* all 10 Wise Decisions!

SPEED BUMPS

Your life is not lived in a bubble. Friends, family, and colleagues surround your dining interactions. Blessed are you if it is so.

When your dining routine is altered by other people, imagine a road sign in front of you: *Speed bump! Slow down!*

Make the decision to finesse your way gracefully through the situation. Do you really want to be the person who takes such extreme diet measures that nobody wants to be around you? Why not choose joy and a little flexibility?

Speed bumps are *not* an ideal time to lose, but they are a *perfect opportunity* to lean into weight loss in a relaxed way without compromising socially. A *social* day is a *practice* day for living thin. During weight-loss speed bumps, your primary objective is only to maintain your new, lower weight. If you'll only slow down a bit, you won't be thrown completely out of weight-loss alignment.

No point in ignoring realities. Do you really think you'll go on that cruise and eat *exactly* as you do at home? When on vacation, I switch my inner voice to that of a loving grandma—indulgent, but never harmful.

Be fearless in *identifying* your upcoming speed bumps, then create powerful advance strategy about what, when, why, and how you'll eat. Indecision is a key threat to thin.

Unplanned moments can be dangerous, so map out a smart, happy strategy in advance!

When expecting company, I make a speed bump-style grocery list which includes special treats that will please *them*—but *not me*. Yes, I choose my *least* favorite brand and style of all snack foods. If we all go out to dinner, I know before I leave the house that I will ignore the bread basket and decline dessert. I estimate my restaurant meal calories in advance. For if I don't plan ahead and *slow down for speed bumps*, I default to old, ingrained habits.

Thanks to my speed bump preparation, I don't have to think much about food during special company visits. We have a blast—with no regret afterward. Our time together is *love*-focused, not *food*-focused. *I do not lose, I do not gain. I do not suffer.*

If my upcoming social occasion is a wedding, banquet, or other group event, I cannot decide in advance *what I will eat. But I can make a much more powerful decision.*

I can decide in advance who I want to be.

Do I want to be a weak-willed glutton who over-focuses on every bite as if it were the only meal I will eat all week? *No!*

Do I want to be a passive slave to whatever food is put on my plate at the whim of a caterer or by a well-meaning hostess less informed than I? *No!*

> *I can decide in advance who I want to be.*

Is the food sitting on my plate the reason I am attending this event? *No!*

DECISION AMNESIA

I recently came down with a case of acute *decision amnesia!* Thankfully, it lasted only two days. It happened during a relative's reluctant move from house to apartment—a big job that lasted two full days and required an eight-member team of family, friends, and paid workers. Exhausted and sweaty, we brought in food for every meal. And somehow, during those forty-eight hours, I completely forgot my important 3rd decision: *I will have a thin identity!*

Why, I wondered later, *did I eat so much and so poorly?* If only I had refreshed and read aloud my 10 Wise Decisions prior to that stressful event, I would have eaten very differently. And I would have enjoyed the whole experience a lot more.

You can immunize against decision amnesia. Make sure you know which decision is your personal weak link. Before any stressful event, be sure to *read, write* and *speak out loud* your 10 Wise Decisions. You'll do fine.

CHEATING?

Have you ever described yourself as having *cheated* on a diet?

To say you cheated on a diet is to use a made-up word to condemn yourself for an *alleged* violation of some diet criteria made up by someone else you probably don't even know. Someone who has no ruling authority over you. You cheated? *Really?* Cheating is a big sin. *And I don't think you did!* Your *non-adherence* to another person's so-called rules means absolutely nothing. Please don't throw around that bad word so casually.

Calling yourself a cheater does nothing to get you to your goal. It doesn't teach, motivate, or rehabilitate your mind, heart, or spirit from repeating the incident. The only thing accomplished by this accusation is to slam shut your confidence. Please never use that word again!

Just because you didn't eat exactly according to the way you (*or they*) planned, does not mean you *cheated*. Cheated on what? A diet is *your* plan for *your* body—and *yours* to change.

You *diverted*. There are reasons. Something was amiss, not quite right: in the plan itself, in its compatibility with your lifestyle, or due to something else going on in your body, emotions, mind, or spirit. *Accusing yourself of cheating on a diet keeps you from learning about who you are and what you need.* Wouldn't it be more valuable to gently explore the reason for the *diversion* than to throw around self-accusations?

Please do not assassinate your character. You are not a cheater. Please never say that ugly, libelous word again!

There is a better way to provide self-support. Do you want to expose the gap between what you hoped for and what actually happened? Use the delightful tool of forensics!

FORENSICS

Watch the film from Sunday's game...

When I've fumbled or gained a few pounds, I don't get upset. I get powerful. I apply *forensics*, the use of scientific methods to solve a crime.

Wait! You say. *Why make such a fuss when things have not gone so well?* Because for you and I, things have *"not gone so well"* for a long, long time. Food fumbling was our way of life before.

Though my food fumbles are now less frequent, I still want to learn from them. I want to "watch the film," to isolate my actions, and *understand* my fumbles. If I "replay the tape from Sunday's game," I can learn new strategies to outmaneuver *future* fumbles. Forensics gives me a *framework* to make a smart and different game plan before the next game. As I strategize and practice, as I adjust my plays, I stay thin. Forensics is fabulous!

I don't want to live my life by default. There is too much "fault" in my default. I want to live by design.

Forensics offers a non-threatening formula to figure out why you didn't love and protect yourself in a particular instance; why you allowed too much food in.

Forensics is cool, calm, and curious. It doesn't accuse and it doesn't condemn. It is pleasant and warm, detached and analytical. If forensics had a facial expression, it would be an empathetic smile.

Forensics is *not* warfare against you. Forensics is totally on your team. It's where you and your great forensic mind team up together to *out*-fox the *out*side *stressors* that caused your fumble. It's not an act of self-abasement or despair. Forensics is fun and *interesting*. You warmly coax out of yourself how you really felt about the fumble. It's cheerful detective work. Actor Peter Falk, who played Detective Colombo on a 1970's television series, is a wonderful forensic role model.

A crime was committed against you—by you. In this "crime," you are both *perpetrator* and *victim*. How and why did this happen? What was missing? What was the true state of your mind, heart, and spirit at the time? (*Hint*: Your prayer journal is a treasure trove for clues about the fumble.)

Be generous of heart when you miss the mark. Dig pleasantly for the hidden triggers that caused you to overeat. Because you do know it wasn't the *situation* that caused the fumble; it was your *reaction* to the situation. Aha! God bless forensics!

> *Thin is a package deal that includes the absence of shame. Thin really is an enhanced way of loving yourself.*

Please remember that when doing forensics, don't talk to yourself like a prosecuting attorney! Be tender, open, and accepting. Dear one, do not rush yourself into a defensive response. Forensics isn't about guilt or sorrow; it's about adding yet another layer of *proactive* empowerment to your *increasingly steely core!*

Forensics will help immunize you against all sorts of outside threats to the thin life you want and deserve. Imperfect *you* will make an imperfect *food choice* now and then. Understanding what happened allows you to plan for a *different outcome next time.*

When you falter, when you fumble, please don't lose heart. Don't give up! *True thin* is about *freedom* and choices; *an ease* of being, doing, and responding. *Thin* is a package deal that includes the absence of shame. *Thin really is an enhanced way of loving yourself.*

Food Marketing 101

When you see an advertisement for food and beverages, how do you react? If they've done their job, you salivate. Beware!

Dear one, you and I are being manipulated by expert marketers whose clever influence in our lives is calculated and pervasive.

Why should we get savvy about food and drink marketing? Because their manipulations are directly affecting our weight, our bank accounts, and our lives. As we grow more aware of what they are really doing, we will be more resistant to their tricks and deceit.

Fake Food

I know a talented photographer whose job is to create well-staged scenes of irresistibly gorgeous food. Her photo shoots produce images that would make a foodie swoon. But you would not—you *could not*—eat the food in her photos.

How does she make it all look so perfect, so mouth-wateringly compelling? Varnish. She sprays the food with shellac.

Yes, dear one, there is a reason the food from *your* kitchen never appears quite as magnificent as what you see in *theirs*. What you see in advertisements has been manipulated—to *manipulate you* into craving it.

Sometimes this food isn't even edible. And sometimes, *it isn't even food!* Imagine my astonishment to learn that certain foods photograph more beautifully *if slightly rotted*. Then there's that illegal practice of placing marbles in a bowl of soup to falsify fullness in the bowl. How horrifying that you and I have actually *salivated* over varnished food, rotted food, or food with marbles in it!

Food marketing is about much more than using digitally enhanced photography to stimulate our senses.

One day I found myself driving behind a Pepperidge Farm truck that showed a huge and truly magnificent-looking plate of Milano cookies. They seemed almost … well, *heavenly!* The cookies were atop an ethereal, cloud-like cookie holder. It took me a minute to make the heaven-connection, but believe me, *they knew I would.*

When you see a billboard depicting a food product, understand that it has been carefully staged to captivate you at a conscious *or unconscious* level, and make you salivate for it.

As for me, I am on to them. I like Pepperidge Farm products. But when I see an advertisement for cookies, *any cookies,* I turn away. I refuse to be manipulated by someone on Madison Avenue who cares nothing about my life, my health, my dress size, my happiness, or my future.

Probably *the sneakiest* way marketers get us to crave a product is by promoting the wonderful *lifestyle* supposedly lived by those who buy it. You are not sold on the food; you are sold on the fabulous life enjoyed by these other people.

Every one of us wants a fabulous life. But we cannot *buy that life* from a food, a beverage, or a restaurant. Talk about looking for love in all the wrong places!

Buy the product, if you wish… but do not buy the manipulation!

Begin to notice food and drink commercials with fresh, savvy eyes. Most show a laughing-out-loud happy crowd of people who all love each other. No one is left out, unloved, or sad. Why, there's love in abundance all over the place. And energy! They are all out there living exciting lives, and you and I will too, if only we buy product X, dine at food chain Y, or drink beverage Z.

Watch the scene carefully. Look closely at the set-up. Feel the manipulation. Everyone in the pizza commercial is happy and thin. The ads for slice-and-bake rolls show a happy family gathered around the table, as husbands and wives connect via loving glances. And what perfectly behaved children! No issues with report cards or behavior. It's a not-so-subtle cue, but most consumers miss it.

Advertisers draw a devious connection between *life* and *food.* You *must* understand that all they are selling is a *feeling.* And you and I have been buying that feeling. *Buying a feeling* from a skilled marketer!

We are wise to remain aloof to crafty misrepresentation.

Dear one, buy the product, if you wish… but do not buy the manipulation!

Fake Life, Fake Friends

Commercials are choreographed to arrest our hearts. Everybody consuming the product seems to be living the life we wish we lived. But they're not living the good life at all. It's all a fake. They're not really a crowd of good friends, only a group of actors, strangers all, doing a job, smiling and laughing on cue. They are only *pretending* to love and be loved, by a *pretend group of pretenders* who are *posing* as friends, *pretending* to like and respect and celebrate each other, as with animation and frenetic energy, they *pretend to* eat or drink the advertised product.

In the commercials, life is an exuberant mix of food, drink, love, and good times. Nobody is tired, nobody gets fired, and nobody quarrels or gets sick. Nobody loses their house or worries about money. Everybody has more friends than the prom queen, and everybody looks fantastic and feels super-confident. Why, that's what you can have, too, if you eat or drink their product!

But, dear one, you won't get that at all.

It's all a fake. Fake happy marriage, fake kids, fake friends, fake home life, fake happiness. When the filming concludes, the actors return to their true personal lives, which for all we know may be lonely, lacking, poor, sad, unhealthy or friendless.

Then there's this: Some of these pretenders—the trim, smiling, good-looking actors—would not themselves consume the food or drink they are advertising. Remember that for them, it's just a job. *It's just pretend.*

Develop finesse to artfully manage your thin lifestyle. Make the wise decision to *finesse the subtleties of thin* so you can stay thin forever!

My 9ᵀᴴ Wise Decision

I Will Finesse.

Signature _____ Date _____

Next: Our 10ᵗʰ Wise Decision is your "Declaration of Thin-dependence"!

I WILL FORGE

Forge your own personal path to thin...

In the past, you depended on *others* for weight-loss strategies. You leaned on their leadership. You depended on their ill-fitting diets.

But you don't need that kind of help anymore.

Why *borrow* an unsuitable diet designed *by* other people *for* other people? Why live by *their* rules? *You* are the expert on you.

If you find a diet that feels just right, use it. If you can't find a diet that pleases you, design your own! *Design a food plan you love!*

You can create a perfect, livable diet, designed *by you* exclusively *for* you. It will feel right. It will feel self-honoring. *And it will work.*

You'll celebrate *perfect imperfection* from breakfast to bedtime. You'll have a *joyous new dessert strategy.* Your emotional moments will no longer be *food moments.* And your appetite will be tamed.

Sure, you'll have a "no" list—*but you'll be the one who creates it,* discontinuing *only* those foods with which *you personally* have a toxic or addictive relationship. You won't play with disempowering foods, and *you won't let them toy with you.*

On a day-to-day basis, you won't think about *diet.* You'll simply make choices that keep you *free from the clingy clutch of food.* Any food that comes with a hook you'll limit, or maybe even drop.

Plenty of tools, tips, and concepts are here to provide tactical support and inspiration as *you establish your own criteria* on what, why, when, and how you will eat.

You're ready. Make the confident decision to *forge a wonderful new plan of your own creative design.*

Peace with Food

Your favorite foods *can* coexist with *thin.* You can achieve peace with food, *with all food*—including dessert.

The eating of something wonderful should not be a stolen moment, but one that's divinely intentional. You can eat anything you want as long as the fork is directed by your will, and is under no other compulsion.

We've grown so accustomed to eating under conflict, with two opposing emotions vying for control with every forbidden bite. We may not even realize there is another way to live.

To *peacefully savor* food is *not* to guiltily devour it.

Dessert Joy

How and *why* we eat dessert is really more important than *if* we eat dessert.

Two Ways to Eat a Brownie

The old way: Skulk into kitchen. Impulsively peel cover off brownie container. Stuff into mouth as quickly as possible. Leave scene of crime immediately.

The new way: Plan with enjoyable purpose and pleasure to include a brownie in today's calories. At your preferred time, go into kitchen. Gaze attentively at brownies in container. With appreciation, pleasantly choose just the right brownie. No matter how small it is, place it atop a real plate; get a napkin, placemat, and something lovely to sip with it. Sit at the table with elegant posture. Pray with thanks that you have the availability and abundance of brownies in your life. Take a small bite and really taste the brownie. Feel the moistness, smell the dark chocolate, and let it melt in your mouth. After swallowing, politely take another bite. Feel the moment, experience the brownie-pleasure. As the last of your brownie is consumed, focus again on your thankfulness and satisfaction with the brownie. If you have time, linger another moment, reveling in brownie-happiness. Then get up from table, whisk away your dish, and leave the kitchen fulfilled, satisfied and with a happy smile on your face.

> *How and why we eat dessert is really more important than if we eat dessert.*

If you do eat a brownie, track it. Not as some sort of "food-sin" or confession, which it *most certainly is not,* but as wonderful documentation that you really can include an *occasional* brownie in your food plan and still lose weight.

Tracking dessert verifies its frequency in your meal plan. I know someone who sincerely believes she is "not a dessert person," but who eats dessert after every lunch and every dinner. Awareness is all!

Our food guilt has missed the mark. The sin was never about the food, but only our magnetized relationship with it. As that element of conflict now disappears, you'll find new pleasure in dining, yes, dear one, even with *less* and *lighter* food. You will be so happy to enjoy your occasional dessert *in blessed peace!*

Peace with food adds *sensitivity* to our pleasure; a markedly different experience than the grasping, gulping, sneaking compulsion-style we had before. Eating is far more pleasurable when we no longer suffer conflict over each mouthful.

Food should not provoke anxiety! It should promote life! You deserve peaceful resolution with food, not an ongoing wrestling match between desire and restriction.

I now choose only what empowers me—and nothing that weakens me. *I don't flirt, fondle, or tease myself with any food I can't consume while still maintaining freedom over it.* My rule of thumb: If I really want something, I eat it—as long as eating it doesn't contradict my 10 Wise Decisions or in any way *disempower* me.

This is how you can experience *food freedom beyond your imagination*—and get and stay thin. Later, you'll wonder how in the world you lived before in such a food-conflicted lifestyle.

Emotionally Charged Moments

Your strategy is simple, and you can do it: *No stress eating. Not ever.*

Think about this very carefully. If you allow a frustrated mood or annoying circumstance to push you off your eating plan, you effectively hand the keys of your weight to an enemy. I regret to advise you that in so doing, you will be tempted unmercifully *in that same way, again and again.*

When you allow *any* incidence of stress eating, *you submit your weight to unseen forces,* some of whom are just plain evil.

Do you really want to do that? Do you want to let your weight be controlled by anyone but you?

Sadly, we, the *un-thin*, have trained ourselves to comfort ourselves with food, to vent frustration with food, to express anger with food, to calm down with food, to act out with food. The equation for our emotional trigger has been: When X happens, Y makes us feel better.

In dog training, a treat is given for a certain behavior until the dog learns to perform that behavior to win the treat. I have a dog, I love a dog, and I know I am *not* like my dog. Yet I had unwittingly trained myself to link undesirable emotions to tasty treats. I had some serious *un*-training to do!

I am determined not to allow the intersection of frustration and food in my life. And for that reason, as an act of fierce, protective self-care and loyalty to self, I prohibit even the smallest bite of food to enter my body if I am angry, upset, or anxious. If I have any negative emotion *at all, I pause from eating until it settles.*

> *I am determined not to allow the intersection of frustration and food in my life.*

This strategy is stunningly effective. You'll know it for sure the first time you get angry—and do not eat. *Wait,* you'll say to yourself, *Something is missing. I forgot… what is it? Something I meant to…?* Then it will hit you: *Oh my goodness. I got really angry… but… I did not eat!*

Just as the thin manage to endure negative emotions without responding with food, you can, too. You are a different person now. You've made some powerful decisions. *Carb-calm* is a dangerous response to anger. You insist on *real* calm, not carb-calm. And when angry, the *last* person you are going to punish is *you.*

COMFORT FROM FOOD

Sometimes you hurt. I know. I do, too. Like you, I need comfort and I need love. But now I know where they come from *and where they do not.* Love does not come from inside a bowl. You cannot extract love from a cookie. I no longer pretend that food is love.

Food has no real comfort or love to give us. It can never fill in for that which breaks our heart. Lasagna can never be our family, our friend or our beloved. *It doesn't know how.* If we give lasagna excess love, the only thing it gives back to us is excess, life-distracting weight, *after which we're just as lonely as ever.*

At emotionally turbulent or heartbreaking times, don't believe the hissed lie within that urges you to grab some comfort from food. Too much food gives neither comfort nor a thin body. But *less* food may surprisingly open *more* opportunity to receive both.

At those times when I am in an emotionally difficult situation, I no longer turn to food. Instead, I repeat these words to myself:

If I am loved by God, who can unsettle me by not loving me?

Sometimes you may have to say it more than once.

By guarding what, why, when, and how I dine, I am *stewarding* my thin identity. I am *loving myself* so that I may wholly and healthfully love and serve others.

Can't I serve others if I am un-thin? *Of course I can!* But I feel *freer* as a thin person. Increased confidence is a booster; it charges me up for wider and greater service. The smaller I get, the more abundant I feel. I'm full of everything rich and good now—*except food.* So I eat honestly, carefully. I eat with thankfulness and with love for God *and for myself.* Each deliberate food choice becomes another victory, another reason to smile.

With a mature mind and a thin figure, I'm packed with new power and purpose. I'm exhilarated! Consider me armed and dangerous... for good. *You will be, too.*

Lovely Hunger

Why do we fear this most natural and healthful part of the body cycle? Why do we regard it as an alien condition? In our food-focused, *obsessively chewing society,* we act as if hunger is the enemy. Hunger seems so *unfamiliar!* But hunger is a *natural part of the body cycle.* It's not a symptom of impending disaster. *Not for us.*

One reason we fear hunger is because the *type* we usually experience is a blood-sugar-based crash that affects our nervous system. *But normal, healthful hunger,* the type that originates from a stomach that has *slowly* been digested and emptied of its protein-based food source, is a lovely thing. You need not fear hunger.

See how little you can eat and be strong, healthy, vigorous and *happy.* Overcome your fear of hunger. *Make a game out of eating less.* Be wildly creative in *what* you eat and *when* you eat. Your palate will be refreshed by a new lightness of eating.

Make a game out of eating less.

Entrapment Foods

You know the snares in your eating. You know those foods you wish you had the strength to leave behind. There are certain foods that block your freedom to be thin if you allow them entry into your body. *I cannot tell you what they are, because your entrapment foods are most likely different from mine.*

My entrapment food is ice cream.

I can have it if I wish, but somehow, it never feels like victory when I do. Though a small portion is not a *diet-buster*, I feel *busted* if I eat it, weakened for having surrendered to its overpowering lure. I don't want to *surrender* to *any* food. And neither do you.

Who says you can't resist a certain food? Or that you were destined to be overweight? That's a big fat lie. Who told you that? Oh. You told it to yourself. Me too. We've lied to ourselves. We've forgotten who we are.

You thought you were that other person, the one who is out of control. But, I assure you, *you are not.*

Is there any food that seems to exert power over you? That for you, represents a form of slavery, weakness, or surrender?

Be willing to drop that food and never look back. Reject any food that seeks to entrap you. When you take a strong stand against that food, you win battles in the unseen world. You establish *a formidable, though unseen victory.* Create your own personal *No* list. Have the courage to reject without mercy any food that would entrap and hold you captive.

Thankfully, ice cream is the *only* food I have chosen to avoid completely. Do I feel ice-cream deprived? No, the opposite! I feel empowered, a mighty warrior who has discovered and removed a weak link from her armor. It is thrilling to confirm to myself that *there is no food that holds me in its grasp.*

There are a few other foods in my life that do not entrap, but that I like … *just a little too much.* Over these, I demonstrate authority by pre-planning and granting only occasional entry. Kind of a supervised access, always with a watchful eye.

If you want true food freedom, it's best to take a strong stance against any food that threatens entrapment. You might even be happily surprised. After a month or two away from chocolate, I sampled it again and happily discovered it was *not* an entrapment food at all, *merely a well-grooved daily habit.* I was thankful.

Not so with ice cream, which I was naturally eager to try again—until I felt those same old feelings of helplessness rise within. So, I now eat chocolate but not ice cream. Above all, I want to live my life THIN & BLESSED, with the least possible *ungodly distraction.*

Who says you can't resist a certain food? Or that you were destined to be overweight?

⚜

DINING ROYALLY

Who is watching you eat?

In the shared kitchen at my office, a long-time colleague rushed in for a lunch that had been delayed by nearly three hours. As I steeped my afternoon cup of tea, I watched her out of the corner of my eye. She said she was extremely hungry, yet she remained *graceful.* She interacted *politely* with her food. She did not even rush to take her first bite! Unaware I was peeking, she carefully placed her napkin on her lap and gracefully raised her fork.

No matter how hungry, Lupe relates to her food with dignity. She is not the type of woman who would pull a chunk of bread from a fresh loaf and eat it in the car on the ride home. I doubt she eats in her car at all. Even when extremely hungry, she takes each bite *as if dining with royalty.* She lives in refinement and restraint. Her dress size is zero.

Practice refinement. Eat as if you are not starving. Eat politely, even in solitude, with mannerly movements and graceful gestures. Experience a *relaxed relationship* with the food on your plate.

Starting today, *honor yourself in the way you dine, even when you are seen by no one but you.* Set a place setting if you possibly can. Slowly savor and appreciate each bite, whatever it might be, *however few bites there might be. Even a week-night salad is a blessing that many around the world do not have.* The lightest of food can be made surprisingly blessed and appreciated simply by the way you interact with it. Your attitude and approach is truly everything.

> *Starting today, honor yourself in the way you dine, even when you are seen by no one but you.*

Eat each meal with the same graceful, appreciative restraint you would demonstrate if dining with royalty. *Because you are dining with royalty, every day of your beautiful life.*

AT THE TABLE

What size plate do I recommend? A great big one! A large, beautiful plate is the plate for you!

Once again, I contradict the experts. *They* say you should use a smaller plate so you'll think you have more food. Oh, how I disagree! Why would I want to pretend I'm gorging on a heaping, overstuffed plate of food?

A small, overfilled plate attempts to fool a gluttonous heart into thinking the plate is overflowing. It *caters* to an unhealed spirit. It tries to play mind games with sin! An overstuffed small plate is *false accusation* of who I most certainly *am not*. I am *not* unable to control myself, different from normal, deprived, punished or gluttonous. No, not me. I am THIN & BLESSED. Hear it?

We never see huge mounds of food glopped onto a plate in a fine restaurant. Fine chefs presume that you, the discerning diner, appreciate a modest amount of really fine, high-quality food. This illustrates a model of how to dine well, even when at home, *even when alone.*

We of a *thin identity* do *not* need to manipulate our plate size. Maybe the out-of-control person needs to fool themself with a tiny, overstuffed plate. But not us. We live in freedom and normalcy in every detail, right down to our dinner plate.

I know what you're thinking. Without so much food on that big plate, can you handle all that new white space? Of course you can! *White space on a plate is lovely evidence to your spirit of the 10 Wise Decisions you have made.* White space attests to your new control; it affirms you are healed of gluttony and on your way to your finish. It is a confident demonstration that your will is flexed. White space reconfirms your mighty decision to forget your overweight-riddled past. It proves your identity is thin and you are living life loved.

White space is one way to *celebrate* that you no longer need to see voluminous amounts of food in order to feel satisfied.

How to Design Your Perfect Diet

My relationship with food was immature and undeveloped. *It needed coaching, reshaping, rethinking.* I needed a plan that was explicitly defined. But I didn't want to put myself on a harsh *diet*.

Past diets had been unnatural and uncomfortable. My heart was never really in the game. No longer was I willing to put my life, happiness, stomach, and lifestyle on hold. Why add unnecessary suffering? *Why punish myself all the way to thin?* Haven't we, the un-thin, already suffered enough?

Meantime, the self-proclaimed experts were all over the place, each claiming to have a secret new formula, a magic bullet. Funny that no two of them could agree on exactly what it was, except that it was a *"secret."*

I decided to add one more voice to the cacophony of unwanted, *unsolicited* guidance encircling me: *Mine.*

For the first time ever, I would forge my own personal plan to thin. I would be considerate of how *I* wanted to eat. At last, I respected the woman within. This decision was my declaration of independence—*"thin-dependence"*—my first step toward true food *maturity.*

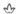

I knew exactly what I wanted. It would have to work *well,* work *fast,* be *pleasurable* and *sustainable.* It would need to represent a short, direct path to *my personal finish,* yet be as painless as possible. Not too much to ask, was it?

I did it.

I forged my own, personal food plan to thin—*and you can, too.*

I love the way I eat. It is so pleasing to me that if I'm away from it for even just a few days, I long to rush back to it. My food plan has *made me thin* and *keeps me thin.* It gives me ongoing pleasure, satisfaction, confidence, fulfillment, energy, and joy. I have finally *defined* and now practice *fidelity* to *my own moderate standards.*

This means I sometimes eat butter and bread—and pizza. I bake brownies (real ones—all the way), and on my birthday

I gleefully enjoy two big pieces of beautifully decorated birthday cake.

Yes, dear one, I eat imperfectly and I'm sure you do, too. *You can eat imperfectly and still lose your weight.* There is no secret diet and no secret food. If we only reduce our consumption and passion to a more sinless state, *we will not have to let go of any food.*

Your best food plan is one that most closely resembles the way you really like to eat, with *just enough creative compromise* to make and keep you thin. *That* is the lifetime winning diet for you.

Something inside you knows what you are drawn to eat. Eat that.

Something inside you knows what you are drawn to eat. *Eat that.* Weave your most preferred foods lightly into a tactical, low-calorie, low-carb food plan that is a pleasure to live with. A plan that is instinctive and natural—not forced.

You are the expert on you and are perfectly able to create a lifestyle of leanness for yourself. You are ready. You can do this. *Design a diet you love!*

Your food list is happily subjective, based on reclaiming your personal control. There are foods you will not allow, because you know they *weaken* you. Other foods you will limit, because they *fatten* you. *You alone have the privilege to determine what, when, and how much.* Nobody else but you.

Are there certain foods you really enjoy but that commercial diet programs scorn? *Declare your thin-dependence. Include them.* Choose those foods you really like and decline those you don't. Don't worry, the trend will change.

The formula is simple—but powerful: Take a little time to think about which foods you enjoy most. Identify which foods keep your appetite at bay for the longest possible stretch.

Overlay these foods against a calorie and nutrition plan. See if you can work them in.

Here's a brand new concept: the idea is to *change* you *as little as possible!*

Please show your food plan to a credentialed professional. Choose that person wisely, and do not hesitate to get a second opinion. If you get ten nutritionists in one room, you may get ten different opinions on best eating practices. One faction insists that you should *not* eat meat. Another says you must eat *only* meat. There's the no-carb crowd, the no dairy crowd, the vegan crowd. *And then there's you.*

Compose *your own diet* in a way that allows you to *breathe* and *thrive* and *be you!* Yours will be different than mine. Just be sure to *define it*—in advance of mealtime—and bring it to life.

Come on, now. You know what you want in a food plan. *Be you.*

⚘

It's also important to identify what you *do not want*. I did not want pills, shots, weird foods, or anything pre-packaged. I also didn't want yogurt or shakes (too similar to ice cream, my entrapment food).

I was unwilling to eliminate any food group or give up what I most enjoy eating. I knew where my snares were hidden, but I also knew which foods represented no problem at all for me. I refused to conform to someone else's standards for my life. I insisted on the freedom to be me—*thin* me.

> *I refused to conform to someone else's standards for my life. I insisted on the freedom to be me—thin me.*

I defined six essential principles. My food plan needed to be *happy, healthy, simple, livable, portable,* and *normal.*

Happy

Food should be pleasurable and feel good to eat. If I have to eat what I do not like, I think about food *more, not less.* I want my mind on God, not on food.

Healthy

I am unwilling to temporarily suspend health to lose weight faster.

Simple

The footprint of my diet needs to be small, very small; my program low-key, my formula flexible. No complicated cooking or shopping. No special restaurants or expense. No additions to my to-do list. Just simple food of my pleasure and choosing to make and keep me thin.

Livable

It has to support my lifestyle, honor my ethnicity, and be adaptable to change.

Portable

We travel. Enough said!

Normal

Natural and appropriate; I want to eat *normal* foods in *normal* amounts at *normal* times.

✧

I make critical demands on any food that *asks* to enter my body. Each must serve my essential principles, must compete with other food choices for my approval, and must multi-task. Each food I select has three big assignments:

- *Keep me satisfied for a long time.* Maybe a very long time.

- *Be convenient.* I haven't got all day to mess around with shopping for it and preparing it. It has to accommodate my preferred lifestyle.

- *Drop my weight.* Weight should fall off my body *and stay off.*

No wonder I'd been dissatisfied with most diets! *I guess I'm a pretty tough customer!*

How To Tame Your Appetite

A significant enemy of diet is appetite. Managing appetite is ground zero in your plan to get thin. Given the nuances of your present appetite, for how long and under what means are you going to restrain yourself from all the food you crave?

Appetite, the official destroyer of thin, has to be managed aggressively.

Through grit? Not for very long! Nobody has *that* much energy. *Not for that.* How can you function if you are rudely interrupted by a loud appetite siren all day long? You cannot endure a howling stomach day and night. If you tremble for food, you'll eat it. And you should.

Managing appetite is one of the most important aspects of

a winning lifetime diet. You are the only one who can guard it. Appetite, the official destroyer of *thin*, has to be managed aggressively. Every food choice must be evaluated in light of its ability to detain appetite!

I needed an *appetite strategy*, and you do, too. I knew that unless I found a way to control my appetite, any weight loss would only be temporary. I wanted the kind of *thin* that lasts forever. I was intrigued. I knew if I could control my appetite, I would control my weight.

I discovered which foods aggressively *stimulate* my appetite and which foods mercifully *tame it.* I was then able to make shrewder choices—those choices made me thin.

The Beverage of Thin

My first great find turned out to be *the most*-effective, *least*-appreciated *non*prescription appetite suppressant of all time. And it was already in my kitchen, literally right under my nose. *Water.*

As a healthful fat-fighter, water is also the least expensive and most accessible choice I know. You already know that without it, you won't live. But did you know that without leveraging water as a natural appetite suppressant, you won't as easily get thin?

Water stalls appetite. You can strategically use it to maximize your weight loss.

Drink your first glass of water before you touch a single bite of food in the morning. This one act seems to happily decrease appetite for the entire day. *Within that first full glass is an amazing gift of fullness.* On the rare occasion I've forgotten to drink my first pre-breakfast glass of water, my meal was less satisfying *and* my hunger returned much more quickly. That first glass of water offers a whole day's worth of comfort!

Drink lots of water throughout the morning, and especially after exercise.

And make it a point to drink a full glass before every meal. A glass of water before a meal is a brilliant appetizer that sets you up to be satisfied afterward with only a moderate plate of food. A glass of water before a meal is so effective, it should be offered by prescription only!

Make water your automatic first responder to any sense of hunger you feel. It often stalls or even stops hunger. I wonder how many millions of calories are consumed by people who are just *thirsty.* Whenever you feel hungry, and especially right before each meal, please drink a glass of water. Especially if you are fasting lunch, it is beneficial to let your stomach enjoy zero-calorie fullness for as long as possible.

♧

Have you ever thought about your water *preferences?* You may not realize that the temperature and style in which you drink can add to or subtract from your level of enjoyment.

The taste of pure water is a gift we sometimes take for granted; a gift that many people around the globe would be thankful to experience. This is one taste well worth cultivating.

With dinner, I prefer a gorgeous small-stem glass, with a fragrant wedge of fruit. *I sip.*

I drink water before meals and between meals, but not so much during meals because I've heard it can interfere with digestion.

Protein

Protein is another way I've found to tame my appetite. I want to eat less frequently, whether fasting or not. My goal is "no in-between-meal snacking." So I choose foods that stay with me longest. A high-protein meal closes up shop on my appetite for many hours. Protein wears off slowly, gently, healthfully. It's amazing how many hours of satiation you can get from meat or vegan protein. I had little appreciation for protein until I realized that fact.

Fat Grams

We all know that fat grams tame appetite, but at unfortunate cost to your weight. My smart phone's calorie-counting app suggests a reasonable maximum of 40 fat grams per day. One teaspoon of olive oil has 4.5 grams of fat, an egg about 5 grams, and a chicken breast about 3 grams, so I think 40 grams is an extremely generous mark to set as my healthy limit. For appetite's sake, I never hesitate to use every one of those grams!

HOW TO STIMULATE YOUR APPETITE

Carbs

As long as I can remember, my appetite has seemed excessive. I thought it was just *me*. I hadn't realized that *I had unknowingly been doing everything possible to stimulate it!* I have finally pointed the accusing finger at the food group that had been my nemesis for all those *un-thin* years: *carbs*.

The worst culprit in appetite stimulation, I've learned, is simple carbohydrates. Even a few bites of a cupcake would set me off to want more and more. *Carbohydrates stimulate appetite.* Sad but true. Carbohydrates do mostly harmful things for weight loss. In years past, before the food industry sold us on eating all those grains processed in their factories, we ate in a leaner, simpler way. Fewer grains. Thinner population. So I keep mine to a minimum.

But since being *happy* is one of my essential principles, I have no intention of living grain-free, or even cupcake-free. I *like* carbohydrates, especially in the morning. As of this writing, I am not breadless. But at restaurants, I've learned to mostly ignore the bread *basket!*

However passionate *others* may be about going breadless, and however fun it might be to get into an *even smaller* dress size, I just don't want to live my life breadless, so I'm not even trying.

Yet, to shut down my appetite, carbs must be tightly minimized to include only that which I hold most dear, on the least possible frequency. I allow myself one slice of bread daily, at breakfast. Carbs stabilize my stomach and make me feel content. So I've made an overall reduction—not elimination—of this food-group that spikes hunger. I eat grain as part of my overall high protein, hearty breakfast, *then avoid starchy carbs for the rest of the day.* When one is eating *less* of something, one chooses more wisely and enjoys it more.

I've reduced my carbs to 165 grams per day, but I try to eat as few grams as is reasonable and healthy. For me, that is usually at least 100 grams per day.

Carbs hide everywhere, and it's amazing how quickly they add up. An example: fruit and vegetables, a most healthy part of any diet. Three cups of innocent lettuce without dressing has 15 carb grams. A little cup of blueberries has 22, a banana has 30, and an apple has 34. There we have 101 carb grams, and I didn't even get my cupcake!

Every so often, I intentionally indulge in pancakes, pizza or pasta as a wonderful treat. On a daily basis, I eat modest portions of fruit, but I carefully choose the *timing*. I've found it wise to include protein when I eat fruit, *because, for* me, the sugar in fruit is *not* an effective appetite suppressant.

The Sneaky Appetite-Stimulator

It's not just carbs that stimulate appetite. There is another significant appetite stimulator, *a sneaky one:* strong flavors. Too many herbs, too much spice, richly flavored food can create strong taste that is addictive. We condition our bodies to crave frequent bursts of intense flavor. We teach our taste buds to expect rich seasonings, juicy fat, stimulating salt, or syrupy sugar *in* or *atop* healthy foods like spinach, green beans, and even strawberries. The more we add, the more our over-stimulated taste buds expect. Is this natural? I don't think so. I've never met a child who, when handed a strawberry, insists on a sauce to accompany it.

Tastes are conditioned and acquired, sometimes to our detriment. If our objective is to detach from the love and lure of food, we need to remove strong, highly defined tastes that most engage it. Beware rich flavors that hook you into wanting *just one more bite*. Strong tastes from herbs, spices, garlic and onions can *awaken taste buds* and *provoke overeating*. And I've noticed that pungent tastes like garlic and onions make me want dessert!

If you *eat as plainly and simply as you can*, you'll soon find that natural food in its natural state *tastes better and better—as your body gets thinner and thinner.*

My Own Breakfast, Lunch, and Dinner

By way of example *only,* here is the food model I designed for myself. Your model may be very different.

High protein and vegetables. Low carb, low fat, low calorie, low quantity felt right for me. I was told I need a minimum of 1,200 calories per day to be safe and healthy. At first, I wondered if 1,200 calories would be starving, but I quickly learned how to derive full and filling healthy menus.

For breakfast, I always eat a generous meal of about 400 calories. On exercise days, I split breakfast into two parts: a very early breakfast that includes bread and protein, followed by a post-exercise high-protein snack, sometimes with fruit. My breakfast combinations are unique and quirky, and that's what I love about them. I might have tuna salad on half an English muffin, followed by scrambled eggs. Or peanut butter on toast, followed by milk with some protein mix. Blueberries often find their way into my breakfasts.

For lunch, it's easy to keep calories under 300. Many days, I fast at lunchtime, except for some apple juice or broth, plus a handful of gluten-free crackers. I intentionally buy the kind I would have no desire to eat except for stomach stability.

When I do eat lunch, I go for pure protein, such as a half chicken breast, leftover from dinner or a few ounces of low-fat cheese. I generally include a piece of fruit. Honey crisp apples sliced thin are sweet and crunchy. A favorite treat is an entire pink grapefruit, cut into bite-size pieces. I make it quick and uncomplicated. Nothing heavy—*no strong flavors to risk awakening my sleeping taste buds.*

For dinner, I eat at least 500 calories. *I know.* It's a lot! *Isn't it wonderful to forge your own plan?* On the *many* days I go above 1,200 calories overall, I'm not concerned. If I've exercised that day, I can consume 1,400 calories or more without increasing my thin weight.

Dinner is a lovely time of refreshment for body *and mind.* Protein satisfies my health component, frequently fish or chicken, occasionally lean beef. *And vegetables just make me happy.* They are *beautiful,* aren't they? So rich in color, so fragrant. But I have to be cautious with vegetables, because I find it very easy to eat too much.

Beverages

What percentage of your daily calories do you want to drink? Thankfully, I've never been a soda drinker, so that was one less thing to give up. But I've always had a daily glass of wine at dinner. As a woman of proud Italian descent, I never gave it a second thought. But after my 10 Wise Decisions, I was not so willing to allow 126 precious calories of *any beverage* into my thin body without careful forethought.

I sometimes still choose a glass of wine with dinner, but often, in its place, I choose a gorgeous small-stem glass filled with crystal-clear water as my lower calorie alternative. I've noticed that if I make it special and *present it beautifully in a stem glass,* it seems to have much the same effect as wine to please me. Maybe the stem of the crystal glass gives me a visual clue to relax. When I do choose a small glass of wine, I sip with enhanced appreciation, for 126 calories is a special treat.

One beverage I sometimes have midday is coffee with real cream and real sugar. I always leave a little wiggle room in my calorie count just in case.

YOUR OFFICIAL SNACK LIST

Snacking is *not* a necessary activity for the sustenance of life, unless ordered by your physician. When in Europe, I've observed that men and women there do not walk around snacking on food, especially while they are performing other activities like walking or shopping or taking public transportation. They eat only when seated at a table for the specific purpose of eating a meal. And most of them are slim.

If you're going to snack, it's crucial to establish an *official snack list!* Without it, your thoughts waver from yearning, to choosing, to surrendering to all kinds of tempting alternatives. *Best to set boundaries, to remove all creativity from the snacking decision in advance of the impulse!*

Your official choices should be ... *boring!* They should only minimally ease hunger, with *no other gratification.* You want to take your mind off food, *not increase your interest further.* Snacks should *never* be delightful and *never be used to satisfy a craving.*

Never eat any mealtime foods as a snack. Not ever! No leftovers. No doggie bags, no cooked food of any sort. *Even if the leftover entrée would be lower in calories than something from your official snack list, do not mingle mealtime food with snack food—not in your mind and not in your body.* Establishing this protective snack boundary protects your forever-thin future and actually eliminates temptation.The best way to become snack-free is to never snack on dinner food. This is a crucial point! Let your mind begin to form a wall of separation between dinner food and snack food, and it will become laughably easy to be snack-free very soon.

Daytime, I choose a thinly sliced honey crisp apple, a

handful of blueberries, or a few gluten-free crackers. I avoid considering any other more interesting option—and *that in itself has miraculously curtailed my daytime snack desire.*

As I prepare dinner, I occasionally crunch on a few carrots. Yes, I know they contain sugar. Isn't that the point? On rare occasions, I've eaten my side salad.

After dinner, if I have a strong desire for dessert *(which is every night),* I drink a cup of strongly flavored decaf tea, with honey or sugar. Very effective. Occasionally, I'll eat a few strawberries or blueberries. For a tiny taste of mouth sweetness, a cough drop or vitamin C drop with real sugar is great, especially cherry menthol cough drops, which confuse the taste in my mouth.

I try to brush my teeth right after dinner, especially after eating strong flavors like garlic or onions, which tend to make me want dessert *as a mouth refresher.*

My best secret to stop a sweet-tooth, day or night, is to squeeze the juice from a half or whole lemon into a glass of water or cup of tea, and drink it. *I defy you to want sugar afterward!*

Late at night, there *is* such a thing as *legitimate late-night hunger,* and I have it often. We eat a light dinner early.

My most effective late-night snack is an ounce of low-fat cheese. Surprisingly, it also shuts down my desire for sweets, just like lemon does. It feels thick and creamy, like ice cream. For crunch, I include a few gluten-free crackers. Under 150 calories and very satisfying.

For sweet chewing pleasure anytime, I'll occasionally munch on a very small package of plain raisins, which are chewy and healthful and satisfy on all levels.

❧

You don't have to be perfect to get perfectly thin. That's good news—because for some of us, like me, the hours between dinner and bedtime are sometimes a bit of a challenge.

On certain evenings, insistent snack-thoughts persistently intrude. Smiling heavenward, I whisper, *"Lord, every hour tonight that I do not eat, I dedicate to you."* Suddenly, I am filled with a counter-desire: to *not* snack.

The most powerful snack strategy, if you can do it, is to dedicate the time from dinner to bedtime as a fast to the Lord. Try it. You'll actually sleep better, and you'll love how you feel in the morning. The best part is, if evening is when you like to snack, *after dinner counts as a fast!*

> *You don't have to be perfect to get perfectly thin.*

The temptation to snack is common to all of us, yet God continues to inspire us with creative alternatives. The one who created us for glory has an investment in our healthy future. *Our goal of thin is worthy.* When we are tempted to snack, we're smart to pause and listen for his creative leading *before* selecting *any* food.

Adventures in Tracking

I want a bodyguard to protect my thin identity. So I track what I eat.

I was of un-thin mind, heart, and memory. My history was un-thin. My expectation was un-thin. My default was un-thin. *Thin* did not yet come naturally to me. *You, too?* I knew my only solution was to snugly wrap myself into a loving cocoon of accountability.

I needed to align what I wanted tomorrow with *what I ate*

this hour. To tenderly, lovingly supervise myself: hour by hour, *not* week by week.

My history had been to consume more calories than my body could burn. It would have done me no good to allow seven whole days to pass before accounting for *my hourly urge to taste.* There are sixteen waking hours in a day, every one of them fraught with the possibility of a snack. Too many chances to lose focus and veer off track.

We wouldn't dream of giving a toddler free and open access to anything they want for sixteen hours without supervision. When it comes to appropriate and godly weight management, I am still a toddler. What to do? Exactly how does one provide hourly self-supervision for sixteen hours each day? *By tracking.*

Tracking is *not* how I bind myself. It's how I *protect* myself. I lack experience in thin eating. It would be easy for me to wander into excess. *I don't want to go there.* If I were driving in the fast lane on an interstate highway, would I not track my speedometer? Well, my lifestyle is lived in the fast lane, too. So my best bet is to keep an eye on the gauge.

When I measure, for example, the dab of olive oil or butter before it goes into the pan, it is part of how I practice living in my thin identity, which I cherish. Measuring is a cozy symbols that I love myself and care for my body, which is home to my spirit.

I am continually surprised by the large number of calories that seem to lurk *everywhere,* even in the healthy foods I love. It's easy to consume a whole lot of them in a day without even feeling like I ate very much. Little things become big things if untracked.

Those few extra seconds it takes to note the quantity of higher-calorie or higher-fat food defines a gentle border to separate my body from accidental or unconscious patterns of un-thin behavior.

I wouldn't dream of writing checks without *recording them in my check register.* I might overspend. It's the same with calories. None of us thinks we spend —or eat—as much as we really do.

I use a free calorie-counting app, synced with my tablet and smart phone. There are many good ones.

Tracking is smart, empowering, and fun. It gives me the luxury of knowing I can eat the foods I really want and still get thin. It helps me plan strategically. And if I feel like changing my plan, I do so with no questions asked.

Tracking gives me a default track to run on. It provides a *framework* for thin. *It helps me be thoughtful about thin-living choices.* By tracking, I find I think less about food—because I resolve my questions and options right away. No lingering thoughts. *No musing.*

The latest calorie-counting apps automatically track fats and carbohydrates. *This solved a crucial piece of my appetite puzzle.*

I quickly record everything I eat. My app includes most brand names, and there is a scanner to post nutritional data automatically, right from the package.

My favorite part comes at the end of each day, when I click "complete this entry." It calculates what I would weigh in five weeks if every day were like today. I find it extremely motivating, fun and very revealing.

The first week or two of tracking can be tedious, so allow for a little extra time. But these apps are so good; they remember your food choices and preferences, your patterns, and your entire meals, so it soon goes very quickly. I spend less than five minutes tracking, morning and night, *including* evaluation and planning.

⚜

Planning each evening for tomorrow helps me think less about food the next day. It's a fun, two-minute exercise that lets me virtually mix, match, and *practice various results before I put anything into my mouth.* Then I consider it done. Because I've preplanned, I don't have to make hasty choices the next day.

Tracking Restaurant Meals

I also find it especially helpful to map out a game plan before I go to a restaurant. Otherwise, I tend to feel rushed at the moment of decision, and I make impulsive food mistakes. These I regret later, and the memory of a lovely evening becomes tarnished.

Since I know before I go what I want to order, I'm less influenced by what I see on someone else's plate. Less likely to be wooed by the waiter's enthusiasm over today's *chef's special.* I'm not concerned about disappointing my server! He or she doesn't have to try to fit into my pants tomorrow.

> *If you eat via impulse, you choose your weight via impulse.*

There are two places not so smart for impulse purchases. One is a car dealership. The other is a restaurant. Something tells me you spend more time in restaurants than car dealerships! *If you eat via impulse, you choose your weight via impulse.*

Sometimes I intentionally choose an unhealthful favorite entrée; for example, my monthly hamburger. *These special favorites are not a deviation from my* THIN & BLESSED *lifestyle.* Tracking allows me the pleasure of fitting those special dinners *into* my lifestyle, with absolutely no weight gain.

GREAT REASONS TO TRACK WHAT YOU EAT

- *Tracking gives you the gift of self-focus.* I'm sure you can recall months, maybe years, of hardly noticing the changes in your body, because you were so overly focused on everybody else's needs.

- *It makes obvious what is working,* and what is not. Tracking calories shows you the truth behind your habits. I was shocked to discover the "health shake" my husband had been making for our breakfast had more than 900 calories! No wonder I was gaining weight!

- *It offers immediate explanation* for results you see on the scale. You'll learn the *why and how* of *thin* for you.

- *You will finally see how much you've been eating!*

- *It sets you up to efficiently budget calories* around your own most preferred and fulfilling foods.

- *It illuminates your path.* It's crystal clear to me now that high-carb days *shut down my weight loss* and low-carb days satisfy with fewer overall calories.

- *You'll connect the dots.* You have always known something is wrong. Why have you gained? Your friend appears to eat more than you, but remains stubbornly thin. *You will learn things by tracking that you will not learn any other way.* Your tracked food is your *black box.* It tells you what led to the result.

- *You'll feel in control* of your choices. My eating has gone from utterly unconscious to confidently proactive. I had been operating on a damaged autopilot in need of repair. Now I'm under manual control. *And I'm so much thinner!*

- *You'll see what normal really looks like. Though for now you may need more,* at least you'll *know* when you are varying from normal.

- *Tracking via apps gives you great nutritional feedback* to monitor your health, such as how many grams of calcium or protein you are consuming.

- *It helps you quickly design a menu.* You can look back at what pleased you before. I created a salad that was over-the-top wonderful. By checking back the following week, I was reminded that I had added leftover roasted asparagus with garlic. What a difference that made! I named it "Perfect Salad" and stored it in the app as a *meal.* With one click, I can post it for dinner next week—and know the exact ingredients to have on hand. Makes my grocery list easy!

- *It's fun!* Tracking is really a whole lot of fun!

- *It's a confidence booster,* assuring me that the great meal I had *today* will do me no harm *later.*

- *It grants a sense of security.* Tracking makes me feel secure and contained in a safe and nurturing way. When my calories and nutrition have been accounted for, I needn't worry about the result on the scale. *If I eat right, eventually I will weigh right.*

- *It creates a valuable blueprint.* For a perfect match, a perfect plan, check your blueprint. Before an important event, if I want to look my very best, I review the blueprint of a time when weight loss accelerated. I duplicate the meals that achieved quick success.

- *It adds exercise output* to your daily recommended calories. This gives you win-win choice. You can eat a bit more today—or lose even more. Either way, you win!

- *You'll have a cool, colorful graph of your weight loss.*

- *It is portable* and can be synced with your tablet, smart phone, scale, and other devices.

- *It serves as an all-in-one journal* for food, exercise, *and* weight.

The Bathroom Scale: Your One-Minute Coach

To weigh or not to weigh?

Naturally thin people may not have to weigh. But I *do.* I want to know, *right now,* if I'm veering even slightly off my path. I don't want to waste a whole week of effort. I want daily confirmation.

Imagine this scenario: A commercial jetliner departs from Paris for Miami. Shortly after takeoff, the first officer says to the captain, *"I have an idea! Let's not monitor our route for a while.*

After all, we have a nine-hour flight ahead of us. Four thousand miles to go! Won't it be discouraging to look at our instruments so often? Let's wait a while. We can check them later."

Ridiculous, of course. Thankfully, airline pilots continually monitor their status, every single in-flight minute, even on nine-hour flights. They receive *continuous critical feedback* and *make immediate needed course corrections. So why shouldn't we?* Monitoring readies pilots to make instant, ever-so-slight adjustments. Wouldn't that help you, too? My daily status check is a big part of what helped me get thin. Even now, I power-up each morning via the daily accountability of checking my weight.

You are on a joyride ... to a new destination called *thin*. Re-routed from your former un-thin weight destination, you're creatively designing *a new route. Why waste time?* Even if you think your flight to thin will be a very long flight, you are better off with continuous feedback. It will help you minutely adjust and make course corrections every single day. You'll arrive much faster if you avoid the drag of unnecessary delays.

While I sincerely respect the rather vocal contingency of *"don't weigh"* proponents, my response is this: *Not* weighing every day is what got me into this fix. If I hadn't forged a new plan that included *daily* accountability, *I would still be un-thin*. It would have taken too long, been too frustrating, and I would have given up.

I am unwilling to wait days or weeks for critical feedback on the actions I took *today,* actions *I might likely repeat tomorrow if unchecked.*

I am a grown-up. Yes, I *understand* that my weight fluctuates every day. I want to be on top of that, too. I cherish each day my morning *moment of truth.*

☙

We need not avoid the scale. We simply need clarity around *why we weigh* and *what to expect when we do.*

One thing you *won't* get from a daily weigh-in is the jump-up-and-down thrill of having lost five pounds. Weight fluctuates minutely every hour of every day, based on liquid volume, food digestion, and a host of other issues. My weight has more ups and downs than the Dow Jones Industrial Average.

My weight has more ups and downs than the Dow Jones Industrial Average.

But those who weigh daily gain increasing mastery over those variances and we learn how to affect them positively. Charting daily weight trends is actually fun. And it's infinitely more strategic than reeling from the shock of a gain and trying to remember what-in-the-world you ate and how you went *so* wrong.

At one point early on, I stopped losing and began gaining. By daily weighing, I quickly identified that having so many high-carb days, *even though low in calories*, had shut down and even reversed my weight loss.

Daily weighing does not give undue power to the bathroom scale. *Quite the contrary!* It *removes* the power of the scale to discourage me or derail my day. Sometimes it hints encouragingly; other times it serves as a warning. Because its daily movements are small, *my reactions are manageable,* and I can meaningfully adjust my meal plan for *that very day.*

Daily weighing helps you make sense of the mysteries of weight. After a recent monthly hamburger night, my weight rose about half a pound. Thanks to daily weighing, I was easily able to make a quick assessment:

Was it okay to eat my monthly hamburger? *Yes. It is probably still digesting, since beef takes longer.* Will I keep watch on my fat grams and overall calories today? *Yes.* Is it a real half-pound? *No.* Is it a trend? *No.* Will I avoid eating a hamburger the day before I attend an upcoming special event? *Yes.*

WHAT YOU WILL RECEIVE FROM YOUR DAILY WEIGH-IN

An incredible education. You'll quickly learn which food and food combinations work for you—*and which do not.* When I was eating frozen diet lunches, the scale wouldn't move for months at a time. Wouldn't it be helpful to know just how much of which foods you can comfortably eat *and still lose weight?* Daily weighing taught me how to incorporate monthly hamburgers, periodic pizza and occasional brownies into my thin lifestyle and *still get thin.* I learned that beef stays in my system longer than most other food, and that excess carbs really do bloat me and hold weight. I now understand the impact of all my favorite foods—and of exercise—on my weight.

Accountability that power-packs each new day. My morning weight hones *my mission* for today. The scale is my daily *one-minute coach,* shouting praise or caution.

A tuned-up commitment engine. There is nothing so focusing, so revving as seeing the gap narrow between your reality and your dream. When I lost even one new *ounce,* my excitement carried me through that day, helping me fend off temptation.

An early-warning system. I'm thankful for scale feedback that showed me that carbohydrate snacks do not support my own body's weight loss. Knowledge is power. I made a very slight adjustment —and dropped to my dream weight.

Maturity! You become wise about how your body runs, and which foods *make it run best.*

A trend line. I post my weight every other day on my calorie-counting app, which has an extremely helpful graph page. That trend line tells the real story of what's going on and where I am headed.

Confidence! Excitement! You really can impact your results by daily monitoring and accountability.

Countdown to Your 10ᵗʰ Wise Decision

Forging your path to thin is going to feel natural and joyful because in wisdom, you prepared for it. You first transformed your mind, heart, and spirit to receive the wonderful blessing of *thin.*

You've already made some very wise decisions of identity, relationship, and process. Before you make your 10th Wise Decision, let's take a moment to appreciate *how very far you have come.*

First, you made the game-changing decision to finish. Without that decision, your next diet would not be your last diet. But now, dear one, *you are going to finish!*

You made the profoundly kind decision to live life loved. Without that decision, you would still turn to food to provide that which you need. You would miss the chance to learn how to *truly express true love to yourself* by the way you eat.

You made the stunning breakthrough decision to have a thin identity. Without that decision, you would continue to unconsciously drift toward a false personal identity of overweight.

You made the life-renewing decision to forget. And forgive. Without that decision, you would continue to be haunted by un-thin memories, negative self-talk, and expectation of defeat.

You made the empowering decision to flex your body, mind, and spirit. Without that decision, you would be weakened and eventually defeated by strong craving and desire.

You made the spiritually surrendering decision to forsake. Without that decision, your affection would continue to be misdirected, and you would miss many diet mercies.

You made the high-five decision to make it fun. Without that decision, weight loss would be struggle of dreariness and deprivation, instead of a constant celebration of engaging, laugh-out-loud wins.

You made the courageous spiritual decision to fast. Without that decision, you would still be in bondage to an unbroken, possibly generational stronghold of food in your life.

You made the creatively graceful decision to finesse. Without that decision, you would be stumped by the first hiccup in your plan.

⚜

It's a brand new day. From a renewed *you* will now flow wildly creative strategies you never dreamed of before.

The fullness of a life THIN & BLESSED is soon to be yours. You are thoroughly well prepared, ready to make the confident, autonomous decision to forge—*a declaration of thin-dependence* that places *you* in full creative charge of your own THIN & BLESSED life. Without this last decision, you would remain dependent on other people's diets that *do not fit* and *do not work*.

With this last decision, you become fully autonomous over your thin weight, now and forever.

Be assured, dear one, your 10 Wise Decisions are going to surround you with everything you need to be THIN & BLESSED.

On your new foundation of peace will dance a new, *authentic* passion as you have never experienced. Your path to *thin* will ignite with a flame that does not waver, but continually renews itself. Strength, love, and holiness will envelop you, and you'll be surprised by lighthearted playfulness in your daily approach.

Your 10 Wise Decisions will lovingly escort you—all the way *home* to *thin*.

MY 10TH WISE DECISION

I Will Forge My Own Personal Path to Thin.

Signature _____ Date _____

JOYFUL ENDING

This past birthday was my happiest ever. What a glorious feeling on one's birthday to *wake up thin.*

I recall a painful milestone birthday, twelve years earlier. On that day, I received a birthday gift that caused me to cry out to God, *Oh no. I've got to do something.*

It was a beautiful outfit from my favorite store. It included a pair of pants that looked as if intended for a child. *Size 8.* No way in this lifetime would I ever get into those pants. *Or so I then believed.* I felt sad … and ashamed.

But *this* birthday, I awoke jubilantly, bubbling with joy. I rejoiced knowing that *I did it! I finished!* Those size 8 pants were given away long ago. *Too big!*

Peace on one's birthday is the ultimate birthday gift to give yourself. A very big present, indeed.

In the end, it was simple, really. I made 10 Wise Decisions that caused my extra weight to crumble into dust, and left me humbly, thankfully, astonishingly THIN & BLESSED.

Many people describe weight loss as a "path" or "journey." *Not mine. Not even close.* A path trudges onward. A journey endures and overcomes.

Mine was a joyride, a joyride to thin.

With each decision I felt a miraculous ascent; steeply up, up, up the mountain, exhilarating my body, mind, and spirit.

Peace on one's birthday is the ultimate birthday gift to give yourself. A very big present, indeed.

As I was weightlessly lifted toward the heavenly sky, I soared high above the bondage of the heavy, food-laden table. And then the thrill, *the downhill rush,* as the pounds released their hold on me. *A joyride to be sure.*

Not that my weight future is riskless. I will press forward, restate, and affirm my 10 Wise Decisions. *And I must never look back.* Paul of Tarsus said it well, speaking to the Philippians about being focused on the goal of Christ:

> I'm not saying that I have this all together, that I have it made. But I am well on my way… Friends, don't get me wrong: By no means do I count myself an expert in all of this, but I've got my eye on the goal… I'm off and running, and I'm not turning back.
>
> So let's keep focused on that goal, those of us who want everything God has for us. If any of you have something else in mind, something less than total commitment, God will clear your blurred vision— you'll see it yet! Now that we're on the right track, let's stay on it.
>
> Stick with me, friends. Keep track of those you see running this same course, headed for this same goal. There are many out there taking other paths, choosing other goals, and trying to get you to go along with them. I've warned you of them many times; sadly, I'm having to do it again. All they want is easy street. They

hate Christ's Cross. But easy street is a dead-end street. Those who live there make their bellies their gods; belches are their praise; all they can think of is their appetites.

But there's far more to life for us. We're citizens of high heaven! We're waiting the arrival of the Savior, the Master, Jesus Christ, who will transform our earthy bodies into glorious bodies like his own. He'll make us beautiful and whole with the same powerful skill by which he is putting everything as it should be, under and around him.

(PHILIPPIANS 3:12–21 MSG)

Come, beloved sister and brother.
Come with me. *Together we can do this.*

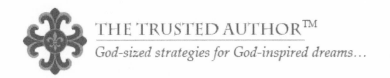

THE TRUSTED AUTHOR™
God-sized strategies for God-inspired dreams…

Write to me at

eb@elizabethbrickman.com

or visit my website

www.elizabethbrickman.com

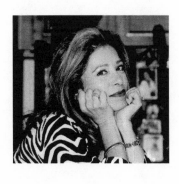

I would love to hear your story and how THIN & BLESSED inspired you.

ABOUT THE AUTHOR

Elizabeth Brickman, CFP®, is a trusted author, a caring advisor, and a popular speaker with a lighthearted and loving communication style. A Registered Life Planner®, she is professionally trained to help men and women identify and live their very best lives. A Qualified Kingdom Advisor™, she is credentialed to provide financial counsel from a biblical perspective.

Elizabeth founded and managed her own nationally successful financial advisory firm for 25 years, at one time managing assets of approximately seventy million dollars for clients in 18 states. She recently retired from active financial management to author books on life management.

Elizabeth's writing style is engaging, approachable, and fun. Her fervent belief is that by aligning mind, heart and spirit, we soar. She motivates her readers to achieve victorious breakthroughs via smart, faith-based strategies she developed to overcome her own personal obstacles, shortcomings and sorrows. Special areas of focus include weight loss, Biblical finance, marriage, and small business entrepreneurship.

Through her publishing company, The Trusted Author™, she offers life enhancing, joy producing, God-whispered encouragement to men and women everywhere.

Elizabeth happily lives in South Florida with her beloved husband, and their lovable, 85-pound rescue dog, Bruno.

NOTES

NOTES

NOTES

NOTES

NOTES

NOTES

NOTES